Do *Safety* *Differently*

By Sidney Dekker & Todd Conklin

Pre Accident Media
Santa Fe, New Mexico

Contents

Foreword   3

Acknowledgements   8

Preface   9

Chapter 1   26
"Do Safety Differently: From Outcome to Capacity"

Chapter 2   59
"When the Work as done is Different From What You Imagined: Do Learning Teams"

Chapter 3   80
"When Things Go Wrong: Do Investigations Differently"

Chapter 4   99
"When there is Too Much Compliance: Declutter Your Safety Bureaucracy"

Chapter 5   134
"When Your Safety People are dejected: Empower Them Differently"

Chapter 6   171
"When You Need To Help Your Leaders Succeed"

About The Authors   206

Foreword

A chance meeting in 2017 introduced me to the ideas of the *New View* of safety. I had just joined the country's largest water utility with a remit to transform their approach to health and safety. With fifteen years' experience as a health and safety leader, I was well versed in behaviour-based safety but was reluctant to keep doing the same thing.

I had a sense that behaviour-based safety wasn't quite 'right'. Morally, it felt like the safety profession had strayed away from our obligations and responsibilities to the essential frontline workers. Organisation after organisation showed the same patterns of dysfunction with safety management: blame-focussed cultures, endless procedures disconnected from the 'real work', and a fixation with metrics that were easily manipulated. I felt resignation and acceptance of how things were in the world of safety.

However, reading Sidney's *The Field Guide to Understanding 'Human Error'* revolutionised my thinking. Rapidly, my understanding of safety was flipped on its head. I immersed myself in all of Sidney's textbooks, published research and YouTube clips. I felt like a new world had been opened to me.

Sidney's writings then lead me to Todd Conklin's *Pre-Accident Investigations* book and podcast. Todd hit the tough topics that safety professionals seem to dance around, offering rare practical advice and ideas backed up by the latest scientific evidence. In a swift three-minute podcast, Todd would pose a question that would percolate in your mind for days, or that you could take back to operational leaders and challenge their thinking. Todd's podcast accompanied me on long commutes and morning jogs and helped me to formulate a plan for my 'safety transformation'.

The *New View* of safety brought to life many practical ideas. New ways to approach just culture; incident investigations; decluttering, devolving and decentralising bureaucracy; safety reporting and measurement; humanising injury management and endless opportunities to leave no stone unturned in applying *Safety Differently* principles. I wasn't alone in my thinking. Many safety professionals I spoke to have had the same experience, in reading Sidney and Conklin's work and being both challenged and inspired to shift the boundaries in their organisation.

With this new theory at my fingertips and an appetite for change among the executive team, I started to formulate a strategy, looking for ways to operationalize the theory and embed this in my organisation. I used both Sidney's and Todd's texts and published research to generate ideas and strategies on how to do *Safety Differently*.

I began by introducing the three principles of *Safety Differently* to the executive team and board and proposing a redefinition of safety, and how we view our people. I took Todd's advice on training and developed a bespoke safety leadership program for all leaders, allowing them to debate and pull apart this *New View*. I used Sidney's *Just Culture* book and *Restorative Culture Checklist* to build a tactical plan to shift from a retributive culture. Frontline workers, alongside the safety team, rebuilt systems and processes to support learning teams, conducted numerous micro-experiments and decluttered the safety management system.

Over a four-year period as Head of Health and Safety, we successfully operationalized Sidney and Todd's ideas. In 2019, Sidney and I filmed the *Doing Safety Differently* documentary to showcase the journey to date and the results we had achieved. Although the documentary offered some insight, more and more safety practitioners would ask me "but how do I get started on doing *Safety Differently*?"

Herein lies the importance of this book. For the first time, the two preeminent thinkers in safety innovation have partnered to provide safety professionals such as you and me, a roadmap on how to get started and a multitude of tips on how to navigate any roadblocks that may arise. This book is the perfect complement to the ideas and theories that have inspired so many to make a fundamental shift in safety thinking.

This book invites the reader to try *Safety Differently*. This could look like taking the ideas and implementing them in one strategy, or one at a time, depending on the appetite of your organisation. Consider the ideas from all angles and layers in your organisation. Where are the champions emerging that might be able to undertake a micro-experiment? Where is there frustration with over-bureaucratization and decluttering that might be needed? Challenge the underlying assumptions about the people in your organisation and encourage a shift from blame to learning. The beauty of this book is that Sidney and Todd have walked the path before us many times over and have amalgamated all of their learnings for us to take forward and implement.

And of course, the road to success is the one less travelled, and not necessarily easy. So, Sidney and Todd offer a shortcut to success by exploring the methodology for safe-to-fail micro-experiments and getting leaders and your safety colleagues on board.

In short, this is a book for practitioners. It is for those of us who want to do things differently, but are unsure where to start. Importantly, this book is not a 'recipe' for the *New View*. Rather, it's a menu of ingredients that you, as the safety professional in your organisation, can pick and choose from to create your personalised strategy. Although the process will be challenging, you have two of the worlds best at your disposal – Sidney Dekker and Todd Conklin.

Every *Safety Differently* journey will be different. But through this book, you can facilitate the basics and kick start a transformation that will bring fundamental change to the way people think about and do safety.

This brave new world is rewarding, transformative and well worth the effort.

Kym Bancroft
Head of Safety, Environment and Wellbeing
Sydney, Australia

Acknowledgments

We thank Darrell Horn and Jay Allen for their support in production and editing of the manuscript.

Preface

> *It was the safest of times, it was the riskiest of times, it is the age of wisdom; it is the age of foolishness…*[1]

Adapted from Charles Dickens "A Tale of Two Cities"

---

[1] Politely adapting the introduction to Dickens' "A Tale of Two Cities" to talk about doing *Safety Differently* may seem like cheating. The juxtaposition of the most horrible things happening while great opportunities exist for change is exactly what this literary device, this Dickensian introduction does so perfectly.

This small book has been crafted for the opportunity to do safety differently. We have combined our experiences and ideas to create a series of important lessons. We want to share them with organizations that are seriously contemplating a change in how they accomplish safety and reliability. We have tried to highlight several important areas to create successful change. While not a complete list, we have selected some of the most common questions we are asked by organizations in the midst of changing safety. We have tried to capture at a high-level these several subjects so this book will help start the conversation and perhaps seed some new practices and processes. The first steps seem to be some of the most difficult steps, so we figured that we should offer some lessons to make these difficult steps a bit easier.

After hours of conversation about what this book should do, we started writing. Neither of us is very used to writing books with other people. This could have been a painful experience, two strong opinions coming together to create a book with some clear ideas to do *Safety Differently*.

It wasn't.

It was the craziest thing; it wasn't hard for the two of us to come together—as we had many times in front of audiences already (some of you will remember *Thick and Thin*, no doubt). Writing this book for you was fun for both of us. We enjoyed a chance to work together for a good cause, and felt this was the right time to help organizations do this important work. It was fun and satisfying to have the chance to toss ideas around between friends. There is no better way to practice the important skill of listening while being humble than to discuss a book on how to do *Safety Differently*.

Neither of us is new to writing books about Safety *Differently*. Between the two of us, we must have some 20 books on this topic. Some of our books you will perhaps have read. You might therefore have some ideas and opinions about the information presented previously. This familiarity will be of great help on your journey to do *Safety Differently*. We are counting on you to supplement the ideas in this book with some additional more detailed readings found in other books available in the world. If you have more questions, if deeper discussions are desired, there are many other chapters written by us and other authors, which are available to give you that deeper information.

No matter what your job or role is at your workplace, we hope that you will be a part of shifting your entire organization towards a new way of thinking about safety. If you are a leader, manager, safety professional, or highly experienced worker, this book will present ideas to help you effectively change the conversations about safety that happen every day. We hope this book will help you and your organization successfully do *Safety Differently*.

Here is what we discuss in the following pages. Use this book as a roadmap and allow this material to help guide your organization on this journey to new thinking about safety. Use this book like a toolbox filled with tools to help your organization make adjustments to practices and philosophies. There will be many changes that need to be made – some simple and quick and others more difficult and time-consuming – just keep remembering that progress happens step by step. Use this book like a gathering of recipes to help ensure you have most of the ingredients in hand as the changes begin to be "baked" into your organization. Finally, use this book as a springboard to even better ideas and practices – we are all in this together.

Change How Your Organization Thinks About Being Safe

In the study of language, there is a long-standing idea called the Whorf-Sapir hypothesis.[2] Whorf-Sapir says that language is relative and that meanings for words don't exist in the words themselves, meanings for words exist in the people who use the words. Doing *Safety Differently* must start with a foundational shift in the definition of safety and reliability for the organization. One of the most important jobs we have is to help the organization change the meanings the organization puts on the word "safety." To *Do Safety Differently* will require defining safety differently in the organization (and by extraction, the people who make up the organization).

---

[2] Whorf and Sapir, although they never published together and did not present this theory as a combined effort, introduced to the world one of the very first discussions of linguistic relativity in 1928. I am amazed by how shocking the idea that people give meaning to words was and is. The power of change often lives in the power of providing new meaning to a word.

We discuss a new way to view safety and more significantly redefine safety. Safety will philosophically change from an outcome to be measured to a capacity that is maintained. Helping the organization use a new definition for safety means we must first help the organization give up the old meanings and definitions. This can be difficult; changing knowledge often causes some resistance in the organization. Giving up the old meaning will be a bit painful at first because there is a lot of past investment (this is often called "sunk cost") in the old meanings around safety. It will feel scary to question something as important as keeping people safe while at work. We have a lot of sunk costs in time, money, effort, and hard lessons to set aside to make room for the new way of thinking. This book will provide some strong support for this transition.

They're not following the procedure!

The second topic in *Do Safety Differently* tackles the worst kept secret on the plant floor. There is a huge difference between how managers *think* work is being performed and how work is *actually* being performed. Because work is filled with complex conditions, it seldom happens the way work was planned and proceduralized. Why this is surprising to managers is almost a mystery. There is very little mystery among the people who get work done—in all types of conditions, daily.

The challenge of this difference between work as imagined and work as done is not about a disobedient workforce. Rather, this difference is more of an outcome of a disobedient work environment—if work environments can be disobedient. But the world has a way of not being compliant with the way we thought that world worked. There are surprises, complexities, unanticipated situations, sudden breakages, and always plenty of ambiguities. Is it this, or is that? Should I wear this piece of protective equipment for this task, or should I not? I am close enough, or not?

We saw a procedure once that instructed workers to apply a 'light coat of grease' to a particular screw-nut assembly. But what is a 'light coat'? That is a judgment call. Judgment calls like that rely on interpretation, on professionalism. But the 'lightness' of the coat might well depend on who is doing the lubrication; on who trained or showed the person who is now applying the coating. Work as imagined says 'apply a light coat of grease.' Work as done gives a range, a distribution of coats, from thick to thin, all under the banner of 'light' in the eye of the applier.

We know (as you know) that when it comes to the performance of work that the map is not the terrain.[3] Although it may seem obvious to you, there is a difference between work as done and work as imagined, this realization may typically come as a shock to the organization. However, as this book discusses in detail, the difference between the actual work and the imagined work is not the problem, it is the reality. This difference is an opportunity to learn; to learn differently. Having the chance to ask new and different questions will suddenly give your organization an entirely new set of answers, of possibilities, of openings and opportunities to improve.

What we think is a much more valuable way to understand this information is how your organization learns about the gap between work planning and work doing. If the work done is not as you imagined, Learn! This difference in both practice and perception is an important opportunity to ask questions differently. One of the best ways to ask questions differently is to use the expertise that currently exists in the organization. That expertise exists in your workers. Who knows better about how work is done than the people who do the work?

---

[3] "The map is not the territory" is a credited to the philosopher and engineer Alfred Korzybski. He used this in an important group of scientific presentations to help the science community grasp the idea there is always a difference between what we think should happen and what actually happens. The idea there is a difference between imagined work and planned work is the same idea, Korzybski simply found a way to illustrate this idea using a powerful metaphor.

Do Learning Teams – uncover the knowledge already possessed by the workforce about these operational gaps to use this knowledge to do *Safety Differently*. Learning teams allow you to leverage the expertise of the workers while engaging the worker in problem identification and solution generation. Your organization will get better answers in a faster way. Most importantly, because these answers are from an engaged group of workers, these solutions are much more effective and sustainable. Learning teams allow the organization to learn differently which directly leads to doing *Safety Differently*.

Not everything goes right

The safest organizations in the world still have failures. The difference between the safest organizations and other less safe organizations is not whether they've had an incident or accident or not. The difference is that the safest organizations in the world are ready for the inevitable failure that will happen. Well-performing organizations know operational upsets will happen and know that they can handle the operational upsets effectively.

As we discuss in this book, to do *Safety Differently* means our organizations must change two seemingly sacred and long-held beliefs:

1. Zero events are the only safety outcome acceptable.
2. Every event has a root cause.

These two ideas are artifacts of old thinking and these two ideas are also wrong. Perhaps more important for our discussion, these two old ideas also stop progress and make learning difficult and less effective. Because our organization holds on to these two old ways of thinking, the organization will not be able to learn much in a new way. To do *Safety Differently* means learning differently.

This book will challenge the old ways our organizations have gathered information about events, accidents and even normal operations. When things go wrong: Do investigations differently. This book will help introduce a highly effective tool to help make this change in your operational learning. Learning teams are just the start of this new learning opportunity. We know your current method of learning must change to better facilitate doing *Safety Differently*.

We are our own worst problem

It is not going to surprise you that many of the complications that we have in getting our work done safely are conceived and created in our operations *by* our very own organization. Over time and with good intentions, organizations often place layers and layers of administrative and bureaucratic formalities upon their daily operations that, and there is not another way to say this, make it harder to get work done.

Is the compliance burden too high? It is time for us to declutter our organization's safety bureaucracy. We live in a world where many of the complications in performing work are self-inflicted and nobody openly talks about this phenomenon. Here is what we know, to reduce operational bureaucracy, we must first recognize our organizations are cluttered with rules and expectations that often serve to provide no more value than just compliance to the rule or expectation.

The futurist Jerry Pournelle[4] coined a phrase for this cluttering of our systems. Pournelle called this "the iron law of bureaucracy" and described the organizational outcome like this: The bureaucracy introduced into our organization by our organization will always strive to protect itself by demanding compliance to the bureaucracy itself. All this is presented to build the case that if we want less bureaucratic difficulties in our work sites, we must first admit that the bureaucratic difficulties are of our creation.

---

[4] Jerry Pournelle was a futurist, a science fiction author, and for our discussion one of the early scholars of human factors. Pournelle coined a series of "laws" he used to describe some idiosyncrasies that exist in organizations. He was far ahead of his time and his ideas are only now, after his death in 2008, starting to gather some traction in organizational thinking.

We strongly suggest on these pages the value of decluttering your organization's work management and support processes. This discussion is exciting because everyone involved in it understands the benefits gained by taking away complications and needless policies and requirements. Change is fun when everyone sees the problem and the direct benefits it can bring. The only real question for discussion is "why has it taken us so long to declutter our organization's practices and processes?" The answer is a part of the discussion. It is found in Pournelle's simple but elegant idea of "the iron law of bureaucracy." We have kept our systems cluttered because we have been told that the clutter makes us better, or safer. Clutter does not make a workplace better. And it doesn't make work safer. It just makes work more cluttered, and it makes the work more difficult. It also widens the gap between how we think work is done, and how it is actually done.

One of the most exciting benefits of doing *Safety Differently* is the permission this gives to declutter an organization's systems and practices. This has also been made more apparent by the recent series of global crises – when workers were divided between essential and non-essential – much of our organizational and bureaucratic clutter was removed by necessity. Does the question then become how many of these rules and expectations did we bring back to operations when work returned to more normal operations?

Doing *Safety Differently* naturally allows your organization to ask some reflective questions about the amount of operational clutter in a non-threatening way. When given the chance to see decluttering operations as a direct benefit to safety and reliability, the need to maintain compliance for the sake of compliance kind of goes quietly away. This is a graceful and effective way to make organizational improvements.

Take care of yourself and you will better care for others.

We purposefully discuss the importance of helping your organization's safety professionals through this transition. Doing *Safety Differently*, while often seen as a refreshing and timely change to the vast majority of the organization, also has the potential to demand huge changes in thinking and practice while sometimes increasing the work demands of the organization's safety professionals. This group will need and greatly benefit from, some special attention. One way to ensure your organization does *Safety Differently* is to set up the safety professionals in your organization to know what it means for them to do *Safety Differently*.

This book recognizes the interesting position where the safety professionals in your organization will be placed while the organization does *Safety Differently*. The safety professionals will be asked to change the conversations they have been having for years with the workforce. They will be asked to move from some traditional enforcement models of safety management to the role of capacity monitoring and mentoring – it is a positive and exciting change, but nonetheless a change.

Safety professionals will also be the front line for this *New View* for workers throughout the organization. Being the front person for organizational change may mean the safety people will feel some of the pushback from this change from certain parts of the organization. This same group must be available to answer questions and provide guidance to the workforce as well. This is not all bad news and gloom, most of these opportunities are exciting and this is a great opportunity to learn and practice new ideas in real life.

An important part of doing *Safety Differently* is to ensure the safety and reliability professionals in your organization are excited, prepared, and engaged in not only their success but the success of the organization as a whole. When doing *Safety Differently* we, by necessity, will need to empower safety professionals in a new and different way.

Leadership will need extra care and feeding

When we sat down to discuss the idea of getting together to write this book, we started by crafting a list of the most asked questions; the most common pain points an organization has in trying out these new ideas. We then discussed what did successful organizations do to create the right environment to make this transition to doing *Safety Differently*? Then from this discussion, we asked: what are the most common threads that run through doing *Safety Differently* successfully?

Well, all those threads run to leadership.

The group that will be asked to change the most is neither the worker level nor is it the safety professional level of the organization. The group that will change the most are the leaders. Do *Safety Differently* really means leading safety and supporting the organization's workforce in a new and different way. The traditional safety leadership skills, skills these leaders have struggled to learn and master, are no longer as effective. The old ways of traditional command and control leadership will need to make way for the new leadership of engagement and empowerment.

This book spends some time on what is the most commonly made mistake in doing *Safety Differently*. This mistake is to *not* give an organization's leadership the time and the resources to lead *Safety Differently*. Many organizations assume a level of expertise and knowledge about *Safety Differently* that simply does not exist among most leaders. If we don't allow leaders to learn how to do *Safety Differently*, where will this new knowledge and different skills come from? Leaders need time and support to lead *Safety Differently* and this time and support must come from the organization.

Using all the kindness and support you can muster, spend extra time helping leaders know what will be expected. Be patient and know leaders will take great steps forward and small steps backwards while learning to navigate the new waters of doing *Safety Differently*. The best news is that once your leadership begins to deeply understand and appreciate this new operational world, you will have the support you need to succeed and leaders will make better decisions that will lead to better organizational and operational outcomes.

In the upcoming pages, we explore these topics in more detail. This book gives us both a chance to share what we have observed as we watch organizations all over the globe do *Safety Differently*. More importantly, this book shares these ideas with you. Use these ideas as you will. Adapt these ideas to your needs. Make these ideas fit for your organization. Try these ideas out on a small scale to see if they will work for your organization.

Most of all we wish you the best of success in doing *Safety Differently*.

Chapter 1
Do *Safety Differently*:
From outcome to capacity

> *"The single, biggest challenge we had in our company was getting our folks to see and talk about safety in a different way. We completely underestimated how difficult it would be to introduce a new way to define safety."*
>
> - An Executive of a Fortune Five Hundred Organization

Safety is having the capacity to make things go well.[5]

---

[5] This foundational idea comes from Erik Hollnagel, one of the great minds and writers in the field. Have a look, for instance, at: Hollnagel, E. (2014). *Safety I and Safety II: The past and future of safety management.* Farnham, UK: Ashgate Publishing Co, and Hollnagel, E. (2018). *Safety-II in practice: Developing the resilience potentials.* London: Routledge.

You may think that this is obvious. After all, if you don't have the capacity to make things go well—in your teams, in your people, in your processes, in your designs—how can you be safe?

But if you look at how organizations measure safety; if you look at what company boards get worried about; if you just glance up at the injury scoreboard at the entrance of your site, you'll see immediately that it's far from obvious. Because those observations tell you that safety is about outcomes. Specifically, safety is the absence of bad outcomes.

Of course, not having bad outcomes is desirable. And if you don't have any bad outcomes, you may indeed proudly declare that you are (or, rather, *have been*) 'safe.'

But there are a couple of problems with this:

- Not having had any bad outcomes doesn't mean that you're safe. It just means that you haven't had any bad outcomes
- Indeed, the absence of negative outcomes doesn't automatically imply the presence of positive capacities. It could be due to luck, or to smart counting (see next bullet)
- You can help your run of no bad outcomes by calling bad outcomes something else (by putting people on 'suitable duties,' for instance) or by allowing your people to underreport

- Most things go well, rather than badly. Much more goes well than goes wrong in your organization. So, if you're focusing your safety efforts on those few things that go wrong, you're only using a tiny portion of the data available about how your operations are doing.

A Ph.D. student of one of us made an apt and seemingly obvious comparison that helped open even our eyes to the silliness in seeing safety as the absence of bad outcomes.

"So, help me understand this," the Ph.D. student said, "you make efforts to improve safety by focusing on the few negative events – the sorts of things you don't want to have – and then you try not to that again?

That is like trying to understand how to have a happy and healthy marriage for the rest of your days by focusing on a few cases of divorce or domestic violence. As if those few negative instances are going to tell you what you do need to do to make your marriage happy and healthy.

If you want to understand how to have a happy and healthy marriage for the rest of your life, isn't it much smarter to study happy and healthy marriages and learn from those?

It would seem so obvious indeed. If you want to become safe and stay safe, isn't it smarter to find out what you should be doing, rather than investing most of your resources into figuring out (from the past) what to avoid (in the future)?

It's still a long leap from where many are today. You probably know the conversation. Your head of safety says, "We're doing great! Look at our numbers! Our injury rate has gone down from quarter to quarter. We've never been this low, and our safety outcomes are better than those of our peers."

This is a great thing, for sure. Just imagine a workplace where you *don't* worry about hurting people who show up to do a job for you. That would be unjust and inhumane, and stupid, and probably illegal. To put a further point… ultimately not very good for business either.

But—and this is a big but—is a workplace with low incident counts or injury numbers a *safe* workplace?

It turns out that, well… it's complicated.

One of us was sitting in the office of a global head of safety of a large (large) mining company. This company has operations all over the globe, in all kinds of different countries and cultures and environments. The head of safety pulled up a slide that showed the injury and fatality numbers across the company. Sure, they were generally low (as in, single digits), as you might expect from a listed global company that tells its stakeholders that it takes safety seriously. The numbers that the head of safety showed were broken down not just per region or country, but also per site. It was fine-grained data. Without making any effort—because it was pretty blooming obvious—a correlation stood out from the slide. There was a clear relationship between injuries and fatalities.

Except it wasn't what you might think it was.

The relationship was inverted. The more injuries a site had, the fewer fatalities it had (often zero). And the fewer injuries a site had, the more fatalities they suffered. The major life-changing, high-consequence, system-collapsing, fatality-causing safety problems were consistently happening in the sites where the injury numbers were very low. They weren't happening in the sites where the injury numbers were higher.

You may have an explanation for this that works for you and that you may be able to relate to your own experiences with safety in the places where you have worked. To us, in any case, the relationship we saw didn't come as a surprise. But it does raise a bunch of important questions that we need to look at together. Which we'll do in this chapter:

- If more injuries lead to fewer fatalities, does that mean that we should be injuring more people to avoid blowing things up and killing them instead?

- Was Heinrich wrong?

- Is it unsafe to try to achieve zero harm?

- Should we even be looking at safety as the absence of negative outcomes (like injuries)?

- And if we do that, then what kinds of safety metrics should we use instead?

The way to do *Safety Differently* starts to stand out when we pick up on the last two bullets; should we understand safety as the absence of bad outcomes? Or can we move to an understanding of safety as the presence of capacities to make even more things go well? We'll take you through an example that brought this into the light for a big (and not so safe) organization. We run you through some of the data that can tell you what capacities you might want to start looking for in your own.

More injuries, fewer fatalities

We have known for a couple of decades now that the safer an organization becomes, the more their injuries and fatalities are going to pull in different directions. Recognize what it says there: the *safer* an organization becomes, the more inversely related injuries (or incidents) and high-consequence, fatal accidents are going to be. So, injuries and fatalities are not *always* inversely related. But you must be pretty unsafe (as measured by high-consequence events or fatalities) for the relationship to be straightforward.

Suppose that you are engaged in something that is, statistically speaking, unsafe—say Himalaya mountaineering, or base jumping (that is, jumping off a cliff face with a parachute on your back). In activities such as these, the relationship between injuries and fatalities tends to be straightforward.[6] The way you get injured is much the same as how you might die. It follows that if you have more injuries, you will probably also have more fatalities. One predicts the other. One is simply an extension of the other. One can even help explain the other.

A popular way of thinking about incidents and accidents is what we know as the Swiss Cheese Model (or SCM).[7] This model holds us to the idea that injuries (or incidents) and accidents are caused by the same sequence of events. The difference is merely in how far the sequence travels. The difference between an incident and an accident is whether or not the final layer of defense is breached.

---

[6] René Amalberti, a French safety and human factors researcher (and doctor and general) showed this. He ran the numbers on groups of different activities: from unsafe to ultra-safe. When you think ultra-safe, think something like the German railways. The chances of getting in an accident there are about 10^{-7}, or one in ten million. Then there are unsafe activities. Himalaya mountaineering sits around $.66 \times 10^{-1}$, or one in fifteen. Base-jumping is around one in a thousand. We'll get back to Amalberti's work when we talk about safety clutter, because it turns out that the safer you become, the less effect operational safety rules actually have on your safety. That kind of makes sense, but it's a neat thing to know, and important to keep in mind. You will also see Amalberti's work back when we discuss the difference between safety and resilience: it turns out that many of the typical things that can make our work safer actually make us less resilient.

[7] The name indelibly connected to the Swiss Cheese Model is of course that of James Reason. He introduced the first version of the model in a book on human error in 1990. The model went through various iterations, eventually ending up being known as the SCM less than a decade later. The model and all of its assumptions, however, are much the same as Heinrich's Domino model from 1931. The eyes in Heinrich's dominoes have become holes in layers of cheese, and the layers don't topple each other like the dominoes once did. But the logic of the two models—their sequential linearity, their causal equivalence of incidents and accidents—is exactly the same. Not much progress in our thinking during the sixty intervening years, in other words.

The fact that a model suggests this to you doesn't always make it so, of course. Fair enough: in unsafe systems, injuries or incidents and accidents tend to be caused by the same sequence of events. And the difference between them is only in how far that sequence reaches. But in otherwise already safe organizations, that is no longer the case. For sure, lots of organizations have believed for the longest time that if they can prevent incidents and injuries, then they can prevent accidents as well. You may even have been told that if you can prevent unsafe *behaviors*, you can prevent injuries, incidents and accidents.

Leaders often really like this idea. The lower they can drive the number of injuries or incidents, the better the safety of their operation will be. Boards have bought into it too, and often approve incentives or bonus schemes that reward leaders who show that safety performance—as measured by the absence of injuries and incidents—improved under their watch.

It's like the broken windows theory of safety. Remember the broken windows theory? A one-time mayor of New York City bought into it big time. Fix the broken windows, and then the crime rate will drop. Even serious crimes, like murder, will go down.[8] For an organization wanting to do something about its safety, it sounds like an attractive (and not so expensive) idea. Because all you need to do to make your organization safe is tell people on the frontlines that they need to behave safely. You can launch a campaign, telling them to care more, to try harder. You can even sanction the behaviors you don't want to see and reward those that you do like to see. Other than putting up some posters, you won't have to do much around the workplace—no design changes, no structural investments.

Except that it doesn't work.

---

[8] 'Broken windows' originally refers to a criminological idea about the norm- setting and signaling effect of small signs of disorder. The broken windows theory in criminology was first tested by Phil Zimbardo in 1969, and further developed by Wilson and Kelling in the 1980s. The theory proposes that the more petty crime and low-level antisocial behavior are deterred and eliminated, the more major crime will be prevented as a result. The thinking behind it is this. Disorder, such as graffiti, abandoned cars, and broken windows, leads to increased fear and withdrawal from residents and others in the community. This then permits more serious crime to move in or develop. Informal social control erodes and allows the growth of a culture where increasingly criminal behavior is tolerated or least not stopped. Particularly in areas that are large, anonymous, and with few other people around, we look for signals in the environment to tell us about the social norms and the risks of getting caught in following or violating those norms. The area's general appearance and the behavior of those in it are important sources of such signals. Whether interventions based on the broken windows theory actually work has been controversial.

Here's an example of a company that wants to show its peers and even other industries that it cares about safety. Workers at one of their plants in LaPorte, Texas were told that they needed to be extra cautious when walking and driving on their site. It isn't clear (and it certainly isn't clear *how*), but perhaps this exhortation helped workers remain safe when walking or driving on the site.

But it didn't keep them safe from a gas release — which had nothing to do with the way workers drove or walked. Instead, the gas release and lack of escape possibilities were linked to long-standing, structural problems that were not within the power of workers to address or solve — even if they had raised issues about it earlier.

HOUSTON — Ten months after four DuPont workers died from a toxic gas release at the company's La Porte plant, federal investigators presented their most comprehensive assessment yet of the chemical manufacturing giant's facility near the Texas coast.[9]

"Safety deficiencies cost four families their loved ones and eroded public confidence in DuPont," said Vanessa Sutherland, the Chemical Safety Board's chair.

On Nov. 15, 2014, a veteran operator opened a faulty valve on a pipe carrying methyl mercaptan, a chemical used to manufacture DuPont's popular insecticide. More than 20,000 pounds of the gas — deadly in even small doses — spewed out. She was found dead hours later, and three men who rushed in to help her were also killed.

---

[9] The portions shown here come from an article by Neena Satija in the *Texas Tribune and Reveal* newspaper, entitled "Report on Fatal Plant Leak Slams DuPont" from September 30, 2015.

In a nearly two-hour presentation, investigators said problems in DuPont's insecticide unit went far beyond lack of worker education, missing details in safety procedures and temporary equipment problems. The chemical safety investigators said the fundamental design of the building where Lannate was produced is faulty.

For instance, stairwells in the unit were the main pathways for workers to move between floors, but were originally designed only as fire escapes and don't have ventilation. One operator was found dead in one of those stairwells. Ventilation has been a focus because fans on the third floor where the toxic leak occurred weren't working. But it turns out that even if the fans had been working, the overall ventilation system had so many problems that the leak still would have caused a "lethal atmosphere," the CSB said. The same holds for the plant's detector system for methyl mercaptan, the deadly chemical that leaked and caused the deaths.

Investigators said there were no methyl mercaptan detectors on the third floor of the Lannate unit, where Wise first opened a valve and the chemical spewed out. Even if there had been, DuPont's alarms systems were only set to go off if the concentration of the chemical reached 25 parts per million. That's higher than federal regulators say it should be. Levels of just 10 parts per million should not be allowed even for an instant, according to OSHA, and the agency recognizes that standard is outdated and should be more like 0.5 parts per million.

On top of that, even if DuPont's detectors did find problematic levels of methyl mercaptan in its insecticide unit, no alarm would go off inside the unit, or outside, either. The alarm is in a control room in a different building.

A worker could enter the building without knowing that a gas leak has occurred and then become incapacitated before being able to react. That is what happened to the three DuPont workers who rushed in to help.

Low counts of injuries or unsafe behaviors do not predict or prevent major safety issues. But there's more. Using a low number of bad outcomes as your safety metric has the following problems too:

- Executives or board members think that they can use injury or incident numbers and compare them across industries, or peers within an industry. But they can't. Comparison between industries or business units is impossible because the measure says something about shifts, not about people or jobs.

- Not only that, the definitions of 'incident' and 'injury' is both variable and gameable. There is little consistency in what is registered as an injury and what isn't. Supervisors, often in coordination with health & safety professionals, will make their call on whether to record a worker's injury or not. And an organization's reward system has a very strong role in helping push these determinations one way or another.

- Also, once you turn the number into a rate (like the total recordable incident frequency rate) it requires a denominator, which is a malleable choice.

- Deriving trends or changes from the measure are meaningless because of its considerable lack of statistical power. With injury numbers relative to hours worked (i.e., injury rate or any other rate) as low as they are, the requirements of statistical significance are never met. In other words, managers or boards saying that they have seen a significant reduction in injury rate, or a significant difference between their injury rate and someone else's injury rate, actually have no statistical basis for their claims. In addition, because of the low power, statistical variations in injury rates from year to year or between companies or business areas, are completely random and cannot be provably related to a manager's or board's actions or inactions. These variations, to put it simply, are way below the statistical noise level.

But...what about the lawyers? The insistence on achieving a low number of bad outcomes is driven in part by a misunderstanding about the legal requirements of executives and company directors. Yes, they need to exercise due diligence and ensure that safety obligations are met. But trying to do that through a single outcome metric is not going to work in the end: it won't protect anybody.[10] There are other ways to show due diligence, ways that are related to safety capacities in your people, teams and processes. We'll conclude this chapter with that. For now, please note that a low number of bad outcomes doesn't protect you very well from legal liability around due diligence. The low number might look good, or so you think. But it doesn't *do* you a whole lot of good.

As David Capers, a Texas oil industry expert who'd been around for decades, told us: "You think it's the LTI that counts, don't you, Lost-Time Injuries? Well, I'm telling you: it's not the LTI, it's the LGI."

Of course, we asked David what the LGI was. He looked at us and then said, "It's the Looking-Good-Index."

How right he was.

---

[10] See for instance *United States of America v. BP Exploration & Production Inc. et al.*, Civ. Action No. 2:10-cv-04536 in the US District Court of Louisiana – the US Department of Justice suit against BP under the US Clean Water Act arising from the Deepwater Horizon Disaster. The prolonged period of operation with no injuries preceding the accident offered BP no legal protection whatsoever. In fact, it may have driven impressions about BP spinning its numbers and/or not really committing to safety and particularly process safety.

A singular focus on metrics can function as a decoy, taking organizational attention away from the build-up of risks and a possible drift into failure in other areas. Underlying risks can then be left to grow misconstrued or unnoticed, as has been recognized by thinkers in organizational safety since the 1970s.[11] LTI is a great example of organizations and boards counting what they can count, but not looking at what *counts*.

Heinrich was wrong (well, he made part of it up)

The name that has become indelibly connected to the broken windows theory of safety is of course that of Heinrich. In 1931, Heinrich was working as Assistant Superintendent of the Engineering and Inspection Division of the Travelers Insurance Company. Travelers didn't just insure travellers; they insured factory owners and operators as well. This made it important for the company to figure out how to help their customers prevent having to make insurance claims in the first place. Could they be told how not to have accidents?

---

[11] Consider Barry Turner, for instance, who published the book 'Man-made disasters' in 1970 and made this very point back then already.

This is where Heinrich was innovative. He can be seen as one of the first people in the history of safety to think critically and analytically through accident causation. At the time, people's understanding of accidents had only recently come out of centuries of thinking about mishaps in terms of divine or diabolical intervention. People had now come to a place where accidents were seen as meaningless coincidences of time and space, without much possibility to start recognizing (let alone influencing) patterns of causation.

Heinrich changed this. He thought of accident causation in terms of a chain (like Swiss Cheese did sixty years later). The chain of causation was set in motion by some condition, and the chain could be broken so that the progression was stopped and no accident or damage or injury would follow. It was an empowering idea and one that could save his company a bunch of money. But how did he know what was in the chain of causation?

He took twelve thousand closed claim files—at random—and started looking through them. The problem was, the claim forms did not contain any fields for filling out accident or injury causes! So, Heinrich started talking with factory bosses and supervisors. What (or rather, whom) did they blame, you think? The workers, of course. In 88% of all cases of accident or injury, workers were deemed to be the cause (Heinrich called it 'man failure,' an early label for 'human error'). So, if you wonder where the figure 80% human error comes from, here you have it. It came from those who'd want to avoid blaming themselves or their systems (which may sound familiar, of course).

But it got trickier still. A small number of accidents had led to fatalities, and a larger number of accidents had led to injuries but not fatalities. Heinrich started to see regularity in there: it seemed (at least from the random files) that there was a rough 30:1 ratio between injuries and fatalities.[12] Could that be extended to precipitating events — those without injury or damage? That would be neat because it would allow him to draw a symmetric figure (the famous triangle). He asked around some, and a couple of his factory bosses thought that it sounded reasonable.

---

[12] The raw data has been lost to history. It is not offered in Heinrich's book. There is no evidence of other analysts pouring over the same data and coming up with either similar or contrasting conclusions. This lack of raw data echoes through the subsequent editions. Even the co-authors of the 1980 edition of Heinrich's book never saw the files or records.

But there was no way for Heinrich to verify neither any of this, nor any data to verify a proportional existence of unsafe behaviors. Because there was no such data. Insurance claims get made when there is injury or damage. No claims get made if there's nothing to claim. So, the insurance records Heinrich was pouring over would have contained none of it. He could not have known how many non-injury/non-damage events or unsafe behaviors there were forever injury or fatality. "The difficulties can be readily imagined," Heinrich lamented three years before his death in the 1959 edition of his book when he was trying to talk his way out of having to explain how he came up with his 'no-injury accident frequency.' "There were few existing data on minor injuries," he wrote, " — to say nothing of no-injury accidents."[13]

In other words, most of the Heinrich triangle is made up.

Does that mean that preventing injuries is not worthwhile? If you want to prevent injuries, then trying to prevent injuries is worthwhile, for sure. But if you want to prevent worse things, then no, it is not worth your while.[14] You'll have to start doing some other things. If you go gang-busters on trying to prevent every little thing from going wrong — like organizations do when they declare 'zero harm' — you are likely to create a greater accident and fatality risk, just like what happened in LaPorte, TX, in the example above. Let's look at this issue now.

---

[13] Heinrich, H. W. (1959). *Industrial accident prevention (4th edition)*. New York: McGraw-Hill Book Company, page 31.

[14] In 1969 more data did show up for a triangle. Frank E. Bird, Jr,

Pursuing zero harm can be unsafe

Of course, pursuing zero harm is a necessary and noble commitment. But trying to run the safety of a company with such a policy can quickly become a bit absurd, and lead to adverse effects.

---

another insurance man (he was Director of Engineering Services for the Insurance Company of North America, to be precise) was interested in the occurrence ratios that Heinrich had come up with in 1931. He wanted to find out what the actual reporting relationship of various occurrences was in an entire population of workers. He analyzed 1,753,498 accidents reported by 297 participating companies. They represented 21 different kinds of industries, employing a total of 1,750,000 people who worked over 3 billion hours during the period he studied. Bird also tried to be more secure in determining the base rate. He oversaw some 4,000 hours of confidential interviews by trained supervisors on the occurrence of incidents that—under slightly different circumstances—could have resulted in injury or property damage.

Bird suggested that removing enough from the base of the triangle could ensure that nothing would rise to the level of severe incidents, injuries or worse. By starting at the bottom, and slicing off something from the side of the triangle, all levels of injury and incident risk could get reduced. Focus on the small stuff, get rid of it, and you can even prevent the big stuff. Bird warned however, that there are many different hazards, task complexities, training levels, contractor-to-worker ratios and such that muddle any conclusions about proportions. All of it can change the ratios dramatically from task to task, trade to trade, company to company, industry to industry.

Some have concluded that all we need to do to improve safety is to focus on behavior. Behavior is presented literally at the foundation of the triangle, the source of all potential trouble. The rest is just a result. Get worker behaviors right, and the rest will follow.

Let's first talk about the absurd bit. Suppose that you are an engineer, a control engineer. You have got a new job, and that is to control the running of a complicated piece of machinery.

As you get inducted into the job, you ask, "So what are my data traces, what are my measures, my indications, that I can use to control this machine?"

The answer you get is, "Oh, your data? Right, yes, well you have one data-trace. It's how often the thing isn't working perfectly. And that is (almost) zero."

And you go, "That's it?"

The answer is, "Yes, that's it. Just keep that number as close to zero, or on zero, and we're good."

Would you take the job? Or walk away?

In control engineering terms, this is called the 'fundamental regulator paradox.' It says that if you regulate a machine so well that it bends your key data stream toward zero, and then you'll soon have nothing to regulate the machine on. You start to fly blind. You won't know what it's doing, and what you need to do. Until it's too late.

That's exactly what happens when we try to 'regulate' the safety of our operations by steering outcomes toward zero. When you get there, or even when you are close to it, what are you using to inform your safe running of the operation? Just keep doing the same thing and hope for the best?

But there's more. Pursuing zero by measuring and incentivizing the achievement of zero can create some strange and adverse effects.

A 2017 study of the top twenty construction contractors in the UK found that 9 had an explicit Zero policy in place.[15] *Six of these companies were operating a safety program referencing zero, whereas the other three included clear statements around zero, for example, that zero was either a target within their wider program or specifically referenced as 'incident and injury free'.*

When the researchers correlated the data with accident data for the period 2011/12–2014/15, they found, to their surprise, the following:

- *There were four fatal accidents for companies with zero safety.*
- *There were zero fatal accidents for companies without zero safety.*

Furthermore, concerning major/specified injuries a similar pattern emerges from the data within the period 2011 – 2015:

- *There were 214 major injuries for companies with zero safety.*
- *There were 135 major injuries for companies without zero safety.*

Could these data be corrected for volume or turnover? It turned out that they couldn't. Even with turnover taken into account, a Zero policy was still an unsafe thing to embrace with respect to fatality risk:

---

[15] Sheratt, F., & Dainty, A. R. J. (2017). UK construction safety: A zero paradox. *Policy and practice in health and safety, 15*(2), 108-116.

- *There were 7 fatal or major accidents per billion turnovers for those with a Zero policy.*
- *There were 6 major accidents per billion turnovers for those without zero safety.*

Taken together, the study shows a 'Zero Paradox' across construction site safety for large firms. As a worker, you are more likely to have a major accident while working on a large construction site operated by a contractor mobilizing any form of Zero safety, than if you are working on a site without it. Zero, for construction on large UK sites, actually means a greater risk of injury or death in practice.

So, what is going on here? An organization enthralled by the broken windows theory and concerned about not wanting to see *any* evidence of unsafe behaviors stops hearing about other hazards as well. It can create a climate of what safety consultant Corrie Pitzer calls 'risk secrecy', in which knowledge of hazards doesn't travel to the right places, and in which injuries are under-reported and incidents remain hidden.

As a commitment, zero is fine. As a policy, particularly one with incentives and rewards around it, it is unsafe. Research has shown that paying bonuses for low numbers of incidents or injuries can be quite dangerous. One prominent safety researcher calls these kinds of bonuses or incentives 'Risky Rewards'.[16]

---

[16] The researcher was Andrew Hopkins, who has written a lot about safety and disasters. His book *Risky Rewards* was published with Ashgate in 2015.

Recognizing these risks, the corporate head of safety of a large national hardware retailer instituted a program not long ago in which workers were encouraged to speak up and report hazards and events. He put in a lot of effort to make sure that workers felt free to air their concerns. He gradually managed to build an environment of trust, of psychological safety.[17] He wanted to show his people that bad news was welcome with him — which he needed to hear it if safety needed to be improved and assured. It worked. After about half a year, the number of events that the head of safety heard about started going up. It seemed workers told us, like Spring. Things started to open up, thaw out. A climate of openness and honesty was budding and soon would flourish.

And then the head of safety was fired.

---

[17] Psychological safety is the shared belief held by members of a team that the team is safe for interpersonal risk taking; that members can challenge, question and disagree without suffering consequences to their image, reputation or career. The term stems from the work by organization researcher Ed Schein in the early 1990s and was popularized by Amy Edmondson of Harvard in the late 1990s. It pulls together several research insights about team effectiveness, resilience and organizational learning.

Because the CEO didn't want the number of reported incidents and injuries to go up. His bonus was connected to the company's safety performance. And that safety performance was measured by the number of reported injuries and incidents. The lower that number, the higher his bonus. He could even tell the company's board that he was concerned with safety and that he didn't like the trend of the past half-year – imagine that, more incidents and injuries! So, he had to act. With the head of safety gone, trust and honesty disappeared too. Workers reverted to trying to ignore their sprains, and patched up their injuries in the restrooms, so as not to attract the ire of their supervisor. A new Ice Age of safety secrecy descended on the company. The safety metrics started looking stellar again. And the CEO got a big bonus.

This is the type of dilemma that we'd love to help you get out of. But for that to happen, we need to agree on possible rigorous alternatives for leaders and other stakeholders to start thinking around.

Safety as the capacity to make things go well

The major shift to make is this: stop seeing safety as the absence of negative outcomes. And, if you are a safety professional or a leader, stop seeing your job as trying to prevent (or rename) those bad outcomes just so your numbers look good. Instead, start seeing safety as the presence of capacities that make things go well. And see your job as identifying and enhancing those capacities.

The question that most organizations yearn to have answered, though, is this: what is going to take the place of their long-held and easily communicated LTIs or total recordable injury frequency rate? As Thomas Kuhn pointed out, people are unwilling to relinquish a paradigm—despite all its faults—if there is no plausible, viable alternative to take its place.

A few years back, one of us was working, together with some students, with a large health authority, which employed some 25,000 people. The patient safety statistics were dire, if typical: one in thirteen of the patients who walked (or were carried) through the doors to receive care were hurt in the process of receiving that care. 1 in 13, or 7%. These numbers weren't unique, of course.

When we asked the health authority what they typically found in the one case that went wrong — the one that turned into an 'adverse event,' the one that inflicted harm on the patient — here is what they came up with. After all, they had plenty of data to go on: one out of thirteen in a large healthcare system can add up to a sizable number of patients per day. So, in the patterns that all this data yielded, they consistently found:

- Workarounds
- Shortcuts
- Violations
- Guidelines not followed
- Errors and miscalculations
- Unfindable people or medical instruments
- Unreliable measurements
- User-unfriendly technologies
- Organizational frustrations
- Supervisory shortcomings

It seemed an intuitive and straightforward list. It was also a list that still firmly belonged to Heinrich's era in our understanding of safety: that of the person as the weakest link, of the 'human factor' as a set of mental and moral deficiencies that only great systems and stringent supervision can meaningfully guard against. In that sort of logic, we've got great systems and solid procedures—it's just those people who are unreliable or non-compliant:

- People are the problem to control
- We need to find out what people did wrong
- We write or enforce more rules
- We tell everyone to try harder
- We get rid of bad apples

Many organizational strategies, to the extent that you can call them that, were indeed organized around these very premises. Poster campaigns that reminded people of particular risks they needed to be aware of, for instance. Or strict surveillance and compliance monitoring with respect to certain 'zero-tolerance' or 'red-rule' activities (e.g., hand hygiene, drug administration protocols). Or a 'just culture' process that got those lower on the medical competence hierarchy more frequently 'just-cultured' (code for suspended, demoted, dismissed, fired) than those with more power in the system. Or some miserably measly attention to supervisor leadership training.

We were of course interested to know the extent to which these investments in reducing the 'one in thirteen' had paid off. They hadn't. The health authority was still stuck at one in thirteen. SO, We asked: "What about the other twelve? Do you even know why they go well? Have you ever asked yourself that question?" The answer we got was "no." All the resources that the health authority had were directed toward investigating and understanding the ones that went wrong. There was organizational, reputational and political pressure to do so, for sure. And the resources to investigate the instances of harm were too meagre, to begin with. So, this is all they could do. We then offered to do it for them. And so, in an acutely unscientific but highly opportunistic way, we spent time in the hospitals of the authority to find out what happened when things went well when there was no evidence of adverse events or patient harm.

When we got back together after weeks, we compared notes. At first, we couldn't believe it, thinking that what we had found was just a fluke, an irregular and rare irritant in data that should otherwise have been telling us something quite different. But it turned out that everybody had found that in the twelve cases that go well, that doesn't result in an adverse event or patient harm, there were:

- Workarounds
- Shortcuts
- Violations
- Guidelines not followed
- Errors and miscalculations
- Unfindable people or medical instruments
- Unreliable measurements
- User-unfriendly technologies
- Organizational frustrations
- Supervisory shortcomings

It didn't seem to make a difference! These things showed up all the time, whether the outcome was good or bad. It should not come as a surprise. Research reminds us of 'the banality of accidents:'

the interior life of organizations is always messy, only partially well-coordinated and full of adaptations, nuances, sacrifices and work that is done in ways that are quite different from any idealized image of it. When you lift the lid on that grubby organizational life, there is often no discernable difference between the organization that is about to have an accident or adverse event, and the one that won't, or the one that just had one.[18]

This means that focusing on people as a problem to control — increasing surveillance, compliance and sanctioning — does little to reduce the number of bad outcomes. But if these things don't make a difference between what goes well and what goes wrong, then what does? We were still left with a relatively stable piece of data: one in thirteen went wrong and kept going wrong. What explained the difference if it wasn't the absence of negative things (violations, shortcuts, workarounds, and so forth)? This is not just an academic question. If you were a manager (or clinician, or especially patient) in this sort of system, you'd like to know. You would love to get your hands on the levers and push or nudge the system toward more good outcomes and further away from those few bad ones.

So, we looked at our data again. Because there was more in there. And we started holding it up against the research that we knew, and some that we didn't yet know. In the twelve cases that went well, we found more of the following than in the one that didn't go so well:

---

[18] Vaughan, D. (1999). The dark side of organizations: Mistake, misconduct, and disaster. *Annual Review of Sociology, 25*(1), 271-305.

- **Diversity of opinion and the possibility to voice dissent**. Diversity comes in a variety of ways, but professional diversity (e.g., compared to gender and racial diversity) is the most important one in this context. Yet whether the team is professionally diverse or not, voicing dissent can be difficult. It is much easier to shut up than to speak up. I was reminded of Ray Dalio, CEO of a large investment fund, who has fired people for not disagreeing with him. He said to his employees: *You are not entitled to hold a dissenting opinion*...WHICH YOU DON'T VOICE.

- **Keeping a discussion on risk alive** and not taking past success as a guarantee for safety. In complex systems, past results are no assurance for the same outcome today, because things may have subtly shifted and changed. Even in repetitive work (landing a big jet, conducting the fourth bypass surgery of the day), repetition doesn't mean replicability or reliability: the need to be poised to adapt is ever-present. Making this explicit in briefings, toolboxes or other pre-job conversations that address the subtleties and choreographies of the present task, will help things go well.

- **Deference to expertise**. Deference to expertise is generally deemed critical for maintaining safety. Signals of potential danger, after all, and of a gradual drift into failure, can be missed by those who are not familiar with the messy details of practice. Asking the one who does the job at the sharp end, rather than the one who sits at the blunt end somewhere, is a recommendation that comes from High-Reliability Theory as well. Expertise doesn't mean ONLY front-line people. The size and complexity of some operations can require a collation of engineering, operational and organizational expertise, but high-reliability organizations push decision making down and around, creating a recognizable pattern of decisions 'migrating' to expertise.

- **Ability to say stop**. Amy Edmondson at Harvard calls for the presence of 'psychological safety' a crucial capacity in teams that allow members to safely speak up and voice concerns. In her work on medical teams, too, the presence of such capacities was much more predictive of good outcomes than the absence of non-compliance or other negative indicators.

- **Broken down barriers between hierarchies and departments**. A point frequently made in organizational research, and also in the sociological postmortems of big accidents, is that the totality of intelligence required to foresee bad things is often present in an organization but scattered across various units or silos. Get people to talk to each other — research, operations, production, and safety personnel — break down the barriers between them.

- **Don't wait for audits or inspections to improve**. This is one that quality guru

Deming found as well. If the team or organization waited for an audit or an inspection to discover failed parts or processes, they were way behind the curve. After all, you cannot INSPECT safety or quality INTO a process: the people who do the process CREATE safety—every day. Subtle, uncelebrated expressions of expertise are rife (a paper cup on the flap handle of a big jet; the wire tie around the fence so the train driver knows where to stop to tip the mine tailings; draft beer handles on identical controls in a nuclear power plant control room, to know which is which; the home-tinkered redesigned crash cart in a hospital ward). These are among the kinds of improvements and ways in which workers 'finish the design' of their systems so that error traps are eliminated and things go well rather than badly.

- **Pride of workmanship**, another of Deming's points, is linked to the willingness and ability to improve without being prodded by audits or inspections. Teams that take evident pride in the products of their work (and the workmanship that makes it so) tended to end up with more good results. What can an organization do to support this? They can start by enabling their workers to do what they want to do and need to do, by removing unnecessary constraints and decluttering the bureaucracy surrounding their daily life on the job.

How much 'more' of this did we find in the twelve cases (out of thirteen) that went well? That is impossible to answer. As said, the 'study'—such as it was—was an opportunistic deep-dive into a complex organization The list above is not so much a set of conclusions, but a set of hypotheses. Are these starting points for you and your organization to identify some of the capacities that make things go well? We reckon they are. How would you enhance those capacities? What can you do to make them even better, more omnipresent, and more resilient? And perhaps you have found other capacities in your teams, in your people, and in your systems and processes that account for good outcomes. What are they? What can you add to the list? With this book in hand, we would like to invite you to compare notes on a much wider scale—to identify and enhance the capacities that make things go well.

Discussion questions

1. Consider the list of capacities that make things go well in the example from this chapter (e.g. diversity of opinion, ability to say stop). Is there any capacity you are missing and that you are seeing (or would *like* to see) in your own organization?

2. The safer your organization or industry becomes, the more inverse the correlation between injuries and accidents tends to become. Why is that, you think?

3. Does your organization believe that Heinrich was right? And if so, about what? Should you try to change that?

4. Safety metrics can amount to a 'Looking Good Index' (or LGI). Who in your organization is trying to (make whom) look good, and for which stakeholders or what purposes? Does your organization measure or otherwise track the presence of capacities that make things go well? If not, what are the obstacles to them doing so?

5. Does your organization have a Zero Harm policy or goal? Is it aware of the increased fatality risks associated with such a policy or goal? What might you do about that?

Chapter 2:
When the work done is not as you imagined:
Do learning teams

> "When you are not getting the answers you need from your workers, it is not a problem with your workers. It is a problem with your question."
>
> -Betty Sue Flowers[19]

---

[19] Betty Sue Flowers is Emerita Professor at the University of Texas in Austin. I highly recommend Ms. Flowers and Peter Senge's 2004 book. *Human Purpose and the Field of the Future*. We like it when two authors get together and share a vision.

If you want to know how work is being done, whom do you ask? If you said any answer other than the people who do the work, then you should step away from this book. Or perhaps take a deep breath and replenish the vigor with which you're reading it. Because you will need to discover, or somehow come around to the insight, that the real experts on how work is done in your facility are your workers. And that is just a start to what they know and all the stuff they can tell you. You'll be amazed once you start listening without judgment.

But, you might protest, I do this already! Our organizations spend great amounts of time and energy resources going to the places within their facilities where the work is being done and confirming that work is being done as to the prescribed processes our organization espouses as the optimal way to do work – safely, efficiently and productively.

Traditionally, organizations audit for compliance. Organizations actively and aggressively seek deviations from prescribed work. Organizations observe workers doing their work to identify "risky behaviors". Organizations walk-down work practices while holding the appropriate procedure in hand, checking each step with the most serious intentions. Our organizations act like some type of combination of a workplace anthropologist and a police officer.

All of this assurance of workers following specific and prescribed work methods is done to assure the work happening is happening precisely the way our organization has planned and proceduralized the work happening every time work is done. Our organizations want work to happen in exactly the way the organization has imagined the work will happen. Through recent history, this formalization of work has become more and more important.

Organizations feel a high need to assure the work being done by the workers is the work that is represented in the organization's formal work control documents. The idea being, we guess, the actual identification and intervention of some type of 'shortcut' or 'creative adaption' will allow the organization to prevent an accident before the accident happens. If the worker would simply follow the process nothing bad will happen, nothing bad could happen.

That idea is crap.

The idea that work is happening the way work is imagined is overly simplistic. It denies the reality that the world of work is a world filled with uncertainty, variability, and constantly changing organizational priorities and operational goals. Performing work is not nearly as predictable as organizations desire work to be – and the act of wanting work to be predictable does not make the work stable or the statement true.

Every worker, without fail every single worker, will tell you the work they do daily is different from the work the organization 'thinks' the workers are doing. Saying that every worker knows there is a difference between work as imagined and work as done is a bold statement. And yet, it is certain that this difference in work as done and work as imagined is real. It is vital information for the organization to capture, and important to recognize.

There is a difference between the work being done in the way organization imagines that work being done, and actually doing work. This difference is normal and the better (and sooner) the organization understands and embraces this difference, the better the organization will function as an effective and reliable facility.

It is surprising to us any organization would still be desperately holding on to the idea that there is one right way to do work. The idea that if the worker would simply follow this one right way, then there would be no waste, no efficiency loss and no accidents. That belief seems to be based upon the simplistic assumption that every day at the work site is the same and that every procedure is complete and encompasses all potential operational complications. But we know, deep in our soul, that every day at our worksites is markedly different from the previous one or the next one. And that no procedure is ever complete enough to actually do work. If you have ever done any type of work at all, these facts become quickly apparent.

Work is more art than science. As much as we desire completely predictable work – work without surprises and variability – we simply don't live and work in a world where perfection happens in complex systems. Workers must therefore be more adaptive than obedient. The work being accomplished in our organization demands workers can translate, problem-solve, and succeed as a normal course of action. We can safely say to any organization the one factor that makes you successful at doing the work you do is the worker's ability to be responsive to the almost unlimited amount of variation that exists daily. This worker responsiveness is awesome to watch – your organization's workforce is quite amazing when all these factors are considered.

Uncertainty is (and always has been) Uncertain

It is hard to imagine a world without uncertainty. The global pandemic has forced organizations to learn the lessons of an uncertain operational world. Every job is filled with operational and production variability – every single job requires workers to adaptively solve problems and make work happen almost despite the process and procedures created specifically to reduce uncertainty. We now know we are not very successful in reducing operational uncertainty as long as we live in an uncertain world.

Given the presence of uncertainty and variability in the performance of work as a reality, our discussion is better focused on what an organization should do differently to best cope with an uncertain world. There is no need to further describe operational variability – operational variability is not the problem. Operational variability is simply reality. What we want to discuss is how to best describe, interpret, and evaluate the difference between work as imagined and work as actually done.

If you want to know how work is really done, ask the worker doing the work.

The world's leading experts in how work is being done in your organization already are on your payroll. You have within the walls of your facility the opportunity to know all there is to know about how work is being done. This information is well within your grasp; all you must do is ask the workers to tell you how the work is being done.

Sadly, it is not that easy.

We are amazed at how little organizations recognize and value the opinion of their workforce about operational and production issues. There are many reasons for organizations *not* recognizing the expertise and information available to them. This information is always within the organization's grasp, bought and paid for by the organization that employs the workers. Many of these reasons are discussed in the earlier chapters of this book.

You gotta talk (and listen!) to your workers

The best and quickest answer is also one of the easiest answers to gather, if you want to know how work is being done at your facility all you need to do is ask the workers how they are doing their work. It sounds easy and it should be easy. Sadly, depending on how much trust and comfort you have in the work environment, it is often not easy at all. We often work in organizations where work execution is kept a secret from the organization. Even worse, many organizational leaders don't want to know how extreme work is accomplished – as long as the deliverable is met, why ask questions you may not to which you may not want to know the answers? We will talk more about "collective leadership denial" of issues that leadership teams often don't realize they are doing.

We can have a long discussion about psychological safety, trust-building and organizational culture – but those topics can be better and more completely covered in other resources. We would highly encourage you to dig deeper into these concepts and constantly strive to improve the operational environment of your organization on a daily, hourly and minute-by-minute basis. Building a strong organizational culture is like owning a puppy, success is a constant effort filled with progress and failure, you are never finished with the work and you will have to clean up many messes left on the floor.

There is a better way

One of the early discoveries on the journey to doing safety in a different way was how successfully we were able to understand how work was being accomplished by actually including workers in the process of learning at the earliest stages of work observation. When you see a problem that you know has the potential to upset operations but do not have a clear understanding of the problem you are duty-bound to learn more about this problem. When you desire more engagement in and deep knowledge about work being accomplished it is time to learn. When you have remarkable success despite many obstacles it is also time to learn.

Using worker-centric learning teams to better understand work in your facilities is a brilliant way to give action to the philosophies of doing *Safety Differently*. Almost immediately personnel will notice a difference in the process of beginning to understand operational pain points. This different approach will be noted; the talk will zoom around your organization quickly.

Learning from workers is fast and accurate

Operational learning doesn't have to be a threat; operational learning can be a tool to build trust and communication effectively. Let us tell you the story of how an organization that one of us worked at accidentally stumbled into its first learning team and how trust and communication unintentionally and dramatically improved.

At the laboratory, we had an event that gained the attention of senior leadership. It seems a new, post-doctoral student worker was doing a field experiment using a piece of sensing equipment that had a rather large battery bank to power the unit for about a year's worth of data collection. While this new student worker was setting up the equipment, he dropped a wrench into the battery box and causes a direct short across the positive and negative poles of these large batteries.

The student worker was working alone and because he was so new to the organization had not yet been to our electrical safety training. The student did what he thought was the right thing to do and grabbed a stick and "popped" the wrench out of the battery box. Nothing happened, no injuries, the equipment still functioned and so the grad student finished the equipment set up and started collecting data. When the grad student returned to the laboratory, he attended electrical safety class the following week where he learned his event was serious, a major risk and reportable. The grad student dutifully reported this event.

The organization was at a loss at how they should respond to this event. The leaders did not feel they should or could punish this person for being honest and yet the leaders felt this event was a precursor to a much more potentially serious event. Because there was this moment of management uncertainty, an opportunity arose to perhaps do something a bit different.

The boss turned to us and said these fortunate words, "I wish there was a way we could just bring everybody in a room, shut the door, and ask them what we should learn from this?"

It was at that time we uttered these words to the boss, "Why can't we just do that?"

He told us to make it happen and that is just what we did. Little did we know, that would be the start of what became a very good habit for the laboratory. It was that day we completely changed the way we did operational learning – and to this day this method has remained an effective response. The organization likes doing learning teams. The regulator is very satisfied with the learning team idea. The results and therefore the corrective actions have greatly improved.

Best of all, the corrective action had little to do with electrical safety and work control. Instead, the corrective action focused on the supervision, mentoring, training, planning and qualification of post-doctoral graduate students working in laboratory environments. We almost fixed one person, but with the use of a learning team, we fixed an entire category of workers who had historically been pretty much fending for themselves in a large and bureaucratically complex organization.

All in all, this operational learning was a roaring success. The stories told about the process ensured we would be using worker-centric learning as a primary tool for operational understanding – and we did from that day forward.

Learning Teams are Easy, Don't Overthink Them

One of the most exciting parts of thinking about *Safety Differently* is applying these new ideas in such a way the organization can observe the change in action. Seeing safety being done differently will help create interest and maybe even excitement for this new way of doing work. Nothing communicates change better than change itself – it's funny many safety programs in the past were quite opaque to the workforce.

A high-level overview of what a learning team does when you are interested in understanding something about your operations is where our discussion will begin. When you have some type of operational curiosity happening in your organization, ask a group of workers to help you do three things:

1. Define the problem
2. Craft some potential solutions
3. Try the potential solutions out – micro-experiment.

Just like in the first learning team example, what makes a learning team so effective is not the generation of corrective actions and solutions, a learning team is a powerful and inclusive way to frame the problem. We have learned that the most important ingredient to effective operational learning is in the actual crafting of the question to be asked – good questions always are foundational to generating good answers. Too often, our analysis is based upon a flawed understanding of the problem at hand.

Solutions are fun and sexy and we have been taught our whole working lives to generate answers fast and effectively. That idea may be wrong; our zeal to solve problems quickly often means that we have not done sufficient analysis and effective problem formulation. If we solve the wrong problem, we will generate the wrong corrective action. Many organizations have very effective corrective action programs that fix the wrong things well. That doesn't mean your organization is bad at solving problems, but probably does indicate your organization is not doing enough to formulate the problem.

What we have found in organizations that are changing their safety programs by early involvement of workers in problem identification is an almost miraculous amount of ownership and engagement of the workforce in operational improvement. Having the workers frame the problem allows the organization to access unusually profound knowledge of the actual work practice – work that is being done during a complex operational environment - and pushes the organization away from the less accurate, perceived notion of the work being done in operations and production – work as imagined, planned and formally captured. This process works well and often produces quite surprising topics for further learning – normally areas and conditions in your facility that simply would not have been recognized by more traditional safety learning and audit systems as important targets for further learning. When you begin the process of understanding work differently you will be surprised by what you learn and the subsequent corrective actions.

The Point of Learning Differently

We know that the traditional approach to work assessment is as comfortable as an old shoe and therefore changing how you learn may seem a bit scary, or worse yet may sound like this will require even more time and effort. Often organizations are a bit hesitant to change learning methods – organizations tell us, if it isn't broke, don't fix it.

It is a bit uncertain when you pass the learning to the workforce; the organization may assume that by giving workers so much independence the organization is giving up some sense of control over the process. It may seem like your organization is giving up control over how the organization learns by allowing the people who do the work to also have their say in identifying problems and operational pain points. In reality, the organization will learn quicker and more accurately about how the work is done. Control does not go away; ownership and engagement get larger – more members of the organization are more invested in creating operational improvement.

Better, more accurate information and higher levels of ownership and engagement seem like real advantages to your organization's improvement process. Knowing more makes the organization smarter. Having engaged workers showing ownership for improvement helps to distribute a shared sense of ownership for the organization's success. These noted factors are real advantages to thinking about and applying *Safety Differently*. Making hard questions easier to understand and the answer is a remarkable advantage for the entire organization. These are big claims to make and should motivate any organization to try these ideas for themselves.

The process of a learning team is captured in the following steps:

1. **Seek potential learning targets** – There is no great mystery in the selection process for learning. Any near miss, close call, near the

event or operational failure with the potential to create some type of harm certainly warrants deeper understanding. At the same time, any operational success is a great place to collect information. What learning does is allow the organization to understand the difference between work as planned and imagined and work as it is being done. Any place where there is operational pain, goal conflict, or misalignment is a place where learning can and should happen. Anytime something happens that places the organization in a position where the organization does not know what happened is where to start learning.

2. **Select or invite a group of workers to be a member of this learning review** - Find people who know the work to be a part of the learning team. Select people who are interested in making the working environment better for both the organization and for the workers. If more people are needed, expand the team to include the people needed to understand the work. If special expertise is needed, bring those people into this learning activity as well. Who needs to be in the team is quite obvious and directly dependent on the work being done by the people doing the work. There will be no great mystery as to the membership in this learning activity.

3. **Schedule two meetings with a gap between meeting one and meeting two** – Find a place to meet and schedule two meetings a day or

two apart to best prepare the group to both identify and solve the improvement target. The use of two meetings is almost entirely logistical – having two meetings allows the group to separate problem identification from solution generation. As we have discussed earlier, the biggest enemy of problem identification is the need to solve the problem immediately. Having two meetings makes it easy to simply put all solution ideas on the second day. This is a surprisingly simple way to keep the solution bias from destroying problem analysis.

4. **Spend meeting one in the identification and generation of the problem statement** – The first meeting, in our opinion, is the most important meeting of the two meetings. Identifying the problem while having the luxury of discussing the problem without the burden of having to solve the problem allows much space for a deeper discussion of the problem and its origins within the organization. Don't be surprised with the group's identification of the problem not being in alignment with the problem organizational leadership may think they have – the problem statements rarely talk about the problem the group was formed to discuss. Learning teams tend to look up and out from the problem and often identify weaknesses in processes well before the problem had become knowable.

5. **Take some soak time to think about what you identified as the problem** – The gap between the first meeting and the second meeting not only serves as a clear division between problem identification and solution generation, this time also provides some time to review and think deeper about the problem. This soak time is normally very productive. Team members often will come to the second meeting and begin the discussion by talking about what was not talked about during the first meeting. This technique is both a way to separate the two meetings that also allows for the benefit of review of the topic.

6. **Spend the second meeting reviewing the problem statement and start generating solutions ideas** – The second meeting not only allows for the review period as discussed in step 5 but also allows the group to go through a review process as a natural function of getting back on topic. This review process further helps to define the problem statement more acutely. The most powerful part of the second meeting is the defined time, set aside to generate creative and potentially effective solution ideas. This second meeting uses the identified problem as a springboard for a multitude of solution ideas – some of which the workers will have been thinking about for years – that will improve the organization's ability to do work.

7. **Have the learning team prioritize the solution ideas** – It is normal to have many great solutions offered up during a learning opportunity like a learning team. Many of the solutions will be effective. One way to encourage a continued sense of engagement is to allow the group to propose a prioritized list of solutions. Have the group determine which solutions should be fixed first, second, and third – Often this periodization is done by asking the group to identify the solutions into one of three lists: long-term implementation, mid-term implementation, and immediate implementation. Normally the organization selects a mix of these solutions. Using the team to help prioritize the solutions is a very effective method to help determine the next steps for this improvement strategy.

8. **Micro-experiment these solutions in a safe-to-learn, safe-to-fail environment** – One of the most beneficial aspects of learning teams is the ability to prototype solutions on a small scale, collect data about the prototype and then move to more effective and sustainable solutions. To allow testing to happen with any hope of success the organization has to make it both a safe-to-learn and safe-to-fail environment. Provide the space, time and resources for these groups to experiment with ideas to improve the work context and conditions. Many of the greatest solutions start with masking tape and cardboard prototypes that eventually turn to fully engineered improvements. This process also

is fun and exciting for the group, not a small benefit in honoring the expertise and skill the workers have for doing work in your organization.

9. **Present information to leadership** – Finally, when the information and improvement begin to take shape, it is time to tell the stories of this learning voyage. These stories are very impactful and important - think of this activity as teaching the improvement story to the leaders so that they call tell this same story to their direct line reporting and their peers. Giving your leadership a story to tell is one of the most important tools to create change – a very important way to do safety in a different way.

10. **Do it again on a new problem or operational curiosity** – Perhaps the best part of doing worker-centric learning teams is these teams can multiply themselves. Once the organization realizes the power and effectiveness of this type of learning, the organization will soon realize the power of tapping into the expertise that lives within the organization all of the time. Tell stories of success knowing that these stories will breed more stories of success.

Change happens through learning

Learning is paramount to change. Change happens when individual members of an organization are exposed to a new way of thinking and doing the work they do. The more individual members who are thinking differently will eventually get to some type of critical mass and the new ideas and philosophies will begin to have a direct impact and the organization will find itself doing safety in a different way. Organizational change is the collection of all the individual change.

Learning is also the most important tool we have as an organization to improve – good organizations are good not because they don't fail, but because when they do fail, they learn from the failure and improve the system, practices and processes that help define work. Very good organizations know work is done adaptively in an uncertain world.

It should surprise no one that the work the organization imagines is happening, is not the work that is being done. Our problem is not to fix the gap between organizational planning and work control and the actual work. Our opportunity is to become better at learning how work is done on a normal day with regular people doing their daily work.

We must understand how work is actually done to be better positioned to create an operational environment where workers and the organization can create a new and different way to create operational capacity.

Discussion questions

1. Why is the idea that your organization may be able to prevent accidents by preventing short cuts or creative adaptations by workers, a crap idea?

2. How large do you reckon the gap between work-as-imagined and work-as-done is in your organization? Does it differ per area? Are your leaders aware of the gap between work-as-imagined and work-as-done? Do they see operational learning from workers about work-as-done as a challenge to their leadership and a threat to their need for control?

3. Are there cases from your own organization where it sort-of stumbled upon a spontaneous Learning Team? Did it recognize and capitalize on the opportunity for learning and improvement, or did it let the moment pass?

4. What would you need to do in your organization to make learning teams an effective standard technique for understanding and improving real work?

5. If you were to organize Learning Teams not to investigate an incident, but rather to look into normal, everyday successful work, which practical trigger(s) could you use for setting up such a Learning Team?

Chapter 3
When things go wrong:
Do investigations differently

- *Change how you define what you want*
- *Change how you learn from yourself and others*
- *Change how you respond to failure and success.*

- From 3 Big Changes... A Book[20]

---

[20] These three bullets are the organizing principles of a book that Todd is currently writing. Of all the observations made while watching organizations struggle with change, these three points always show up in the discussion. Look for *3 Big Changes* soon.

Not everything went right

A small chemical facility had something go wrong.

On a Friday night of a holiday weekend at about 11:30 pm a large chemical tank sprang a leak. This loss of containment event would eventually allow about 300 gallons of a high-risk chemical to be released. The leak was discovered the following Sunday morning when, during a normal walk-around, a maintainer identified the leak and began the response and notification processes. The spill team responded and the leak was isolated, contained, cleaned up, and reported to the regulator.

The facility had a spotless safety record. This event hit this group of workers hard. The response from corporate only served to increase the negative feelings of the local staff and leaders. A loss of containment event that is not discovered for almost an entire weekend does not look good and must indicate some sloppy practices and inattention to safety-critical work. This leak was a black eye on the operations. A better run facility would have identified this problem and never allowed a multi-day loss of containment to go undetected. Heads will have to roll to send a clear message to this and other like facilities.

A team was sent in to do an investigation. The team found the leak originated from a part of the chemical tank that is designed to leak first, commonly called the "telltale" and it is a special section of the tank that is only one wall thick and is designed and engineered to leak first and is a good way to detect a corrosion problem early before the leak becomes catastrophic. Because this telltale is designed to leak first, the tank was designed with a series of recovery pipes and tanks to contain the potential leak the telltale will inevitably have. In reality, because there is this recovery system designed in the process safety protocols no chemicals were ever sent to the ground – not even close.

Daily tank inspections are held every workday. Due to recent business adjustments, this faculty had moved from a 7 day a week operation to a 5 day a week operation. Because this change of schedule had only just begun, the weekend schedules and operational checks had not quite been fine-tuned. In this case, a maintenance worker did a quick and unscheduled (unpaid) drop-in on Sunday just to provide some assurance everything was going ok – it wasn't.

The loss of containment was spotted, reported, and as noted above the spill team responded.

The decision was made to discipline the facility management team by reducing their production incentive payments.

Is this a failure or a success?

It may surprise you to be told the answer to this question is simply a matter of what the organization chooses to see, which details the organization determines are important about this event, what the organization thinks happened.

How the organization responds to an event is a choice:

- In this case study, you can see this event as a failure; a tank lost containment and leaked for almost two full days.

- In this case study, you can see this event as a success; a tank lost containment and the process safety design was ready and able to manage the loss of containment to a secondary containment system with zero loss of product to the environment.

- In this case study, you can see this event as both a failure and a success – a successful failure. A telltale, a purposefully designed weakness to give an early indication of tank erosion functioned as designed and leaked into a secondary containment system giving the organization an early indicator of a potential catastrophic tank failure.

All of these points of view are at least at the simplest level, correct. All of these points of view are potential findings of an investigation or an event review. All of these points of view have the potential for the organization to improve. Yet, not all of these points of view are equally detailed in helping to explain how this event happened.

How the story of the event is told will tilt the scales of opinion in one direction or another. There are no investigations or event reviews without a point of view and the people who review the event outcome after something goes wrong most often choose the point of view, either consciously or subconsciously.

We will revisit the case study in a moment, but first, we should talk about how to do *Safety Differently* changes how event learning happens.

How any organization chooses to see an event will directly influence the path forward the organization will take in response to this event. How the organization responds to this event in the future with corrective actions is directly derived from what the organization thinks happened. Corrective actions are the investigatory outcome and are entirely derived from how the organization chooses what type of response will be used while doing the event learning and investigation activities. What the organization looks for is always what the organization will find.

Often, organizations act as if the investigation and its findings are an outcome of the event. In reality, the investigation and its findings are an outcome of how the organization has chosen to *respond* to the event. And these responses matter. They matter a lot.

An organization's response to an event must be seen as a deliberate choice, hopefully, an informed and forward-moving choice and this deliberate choice will color not only what the organization investigates but also what actions and reactions the organization will take to recover and move on from the event.

Organizations often act as if they are the victims of an accident. Of course, we would agree that an organization could literally suffer from the consequences of something that has gone wrong. To say the organization is the victim, however, is letting that organization off much too easily. The organization is not another victim of an event gone wrong. The organization owns the processes and practices, the systems and the support and ultimately, the entire environment in which the work is being done—and thus it owns the entire system that was behind the creation of that accident. Just like it owns the entire system that is normally behind the creation of success.

The same is true with learning from events: organizations often act as if the investigation will happen to the organization and the organization will be the victim of the investigation's findings. In actuality, the organization should be making decisions that can (and should) guide the organization towards better understanding the multiple complexities present in the context of the event. Event learning is an active strategy towards improvement, not a sentence to be passed down to the board of directors as a verdict for doing something bad.

Investigations learn; Corrective actions fix

We ask organizations across the globe why they do investigations. The answer is often the same, "to prevent re-occurrence." That answer is wrong. Investigations don't change work control, investigations don't fix broken equipment, investigations don't remove at-risk behaviors and investigations are definitely not corrective actions.

Investigations do one thing; investigations provide information to the organization about the organization's processes and practices, systems and incentives, environment and equipment, leadership and followership. Investigations learn (well, the good ones do). It is vital to see an investigation as an extremely important learning opportunity. This opportunity should not be wasted nor squandered; an event has happened and the organization is now duty-bound to learn and improve from this event. Improvement will not happen without learning. The tool we have to do the best learning we can do for our organization is to investigate the event to learn and not to fix.

Fixing will come later. If the organization has done a good job at learning from the event the corrective actions will be effective, clear and obvious. A good investigation writes its own corrective actions.[21] As difficult as this may be to believe, organizations improve when the organization realizes the need for putting the emphasis on learning and taking away the current emphasis from fixing. Learning from events is a data-input challenge and not a solution-output failure.

We would not tell you how to do an investigation. We cannot tell you which method is best for investigating and learning. We don't know enough to tell you what is the best method, the best software, or the best way to investigate. Every event is different and no two investigations are ever the same. We would not or could not endorse one method over another method – that choice must be made by the team of people who are tasked to investigate the bad outcome.

---

[21] This is so strong of an idea that the transverse of this is also true. If your organization does an investigation and is having a difficult time generating an effective set of corrective actions – it is a good bet that your investigation is not yet finished. If corrective actions are not obvious, the investigation is not yet complete.

The best we can do is to discuss how to think about doing the investigation. Doing safety in a different way allows the organization to think about the output of an investigation not as a report on who failed, but as a clear explanation of what failed in the organization's systems and processes to give clear direction as to what in the organization will need improvement. What does the organization learn to get better as an organization? Any method that has as its central goal the honest collection of improvement data will be a good method.

Except for one...

Why Root Cause Analysis seems helpful but is not

Part of the struggle we all share in doing investigations and event learning activities better is the constant pressure to identify the 'root cause' of the accident. Almost all of an organization's stakeholders want a root cause. Finding the root cause of an accident is an attractive idea and we can understand why organizations place so much stock in finding the one, main thing that is bad and then immediately remove that one bad thing. Oh, but if the world would be so simple; oh, if it were only one thing that we needed to remove to make our workplace safe...our jobs would be so much easier. Sadly, there is never one 'root cause' that must be removed or fixed. Bad things that happen in our organizations happen because many small contextual factors have collectively combined in such a complex way that a bad outcome could result in our operations. That last sentence is almost the exact opposite definition of the concept of root cause.

Human beings want the world to be simple. Our organizations (made up of a large group of human beings) want the reason a bad thing happens to be simple as well. However, remember: the world in which your organization functions is far from simple. Therefore, talking about a 'root cause' unfairly and misleadingly builds a false sense of hope that the problems that caused the accident will be simple to understand and simple to remove and fix. This is never true in our experience. Investigations learn many, many things while trying to describe how the event happened. Every contextual factor we don't discuss to support the idea of a 'root cause' could be a vital piece of information needed to point the organization towards getting better.

Traditional Investigations are often limited by Administrative Requirements

Don't let an accounting system or some type of corporate record-keeping system dictate what you will learn as an organization. Far too many organizations are held captive to their administrative record-keeping process. Learning systems that have those terrible 'pull-down menus of causes' limit the way the organization learns and, more seriously, what the organization will learn. These menus allow for trending and tracking of cause-codes but do not allow the organization to learn the complex nature of how the event happened.

There are countless stories of investigation personnel having to select 'the closest code to the actual learning' from a pre-provided list of causal factors. This is frustrating and reduces the fidelity of your learning. Trending seems important; however, trending is much more a part of traditional safety and not a function of doing safety in a different way. We don't investigate trend data to predict the next accident, we investigate to learn and improve.

The most remarkable part of how software systems that limit effective and context-rich data reporting to optimize for data-trending is the fact that these limitations are entirely self-inflicted. Regulators don't ask for this information. Investigators do like this process. The intention, being able to trend causal factors and then predict the future to prevent the next event, is understandable and even desirable. The practice forces the classification of events into broad, non-meaningful categories that are actually not helpful and absolutely offer no predictability for future failure prevention.

The benefits of investigating differently

Perhaps the most profound and noticeable change to an organization's safety program as the organization ventures towards a new approach to safety and reliability is found in the learning outcomes generated in *New View* investigations. Our traditional investigations seem to have mostly been done to determine who failed and to quickly offer corrective action. Investigations were not seen as places to learn new information about the organization's work processes and practices. Investigations tended to seek the place where some type of deviation from expected behavior or process was supposed to happen and then determine that absence of the correct action as the cause.

Investigations in the old way of thinking were truly quick and dirty: figure out what went wrong and fire or fix the person who did not do the right thing. Our organizations did investigations (it sometimes makes us blush to still call them that…), but the actual learning value was quite low – and seemed to be getting lower and lower. With the advent of software systems, investigations became an exercise in filling in the right paperwork; the right way in the right format. Few, if any organizations revisited investigations after the investigation was completed for either learning value or a check on the quality of the work.

Interestingly, it seems that we didn't know the investigations we were doing were not very helpful. When you measure the quality of the investigation by getting it done on time and in the right format, our organizations did not spend a lot of time thinking about what this meant for actually doing the work. When you deliberately limit the amount of information that can be discussed about context, local rationale and work mindset, it is no surprise that our traditional investigations read more like a police report and less like a learning tool. Investigation work was seen as more of a formality and less of an improvement opportunity.

Investigating and learning from events in a different way has opened up the scope of the events. Where once we were almost entirely limited to look deeply into the event, our teams are now much more likely to look out from the event and to determine the entire context of the work environment to understand the complex nature of the work being done, and specifically, the event in question. Suddenly, asking the local rationale question, "what was going on that made these workers believe the decisions they made were the right decisions for the context of this work?" is a normal part of doing event learning.

With more emphasis on learning and less emphasis on blame, the discussion of the event moves to a much richer understanding of how this event could have created such an unwanted outcome. Moving from asking, "Who failed?" to the much more important question of "What failed?" is a seismic shift in thinking in the investigation world. It is hard to fully describe how this simple change from who to what has improved our operational learning. It is safe to say the investigation work being done now is so much better than the investigations of the old, traditional days.

Learning differently allows for worker error. Knowing workers are not perfect, that mistakes happen all the time while doing both successful work and while occasionally having unwanted outcomes has allowed the investigation to go beyond determining cause and fault. In a way, this allowed our organizations to actually do event learning to learn and analyze the event information – to seek places in the work where processes collide and workers must adapt. Having the permission to see a mistake as normal and non-causal allows the event learning to move much deeper into the actual work execution information.

Learning beyond traditional investigations helps the organization discover improvement opportunities that have always been in the work, but were not able to be uncovered using only the old view. We have always known there is more to the story of an event than the worker not following some rule; we were never given a way to legitimately discuss these issues – until organizations started experimenting with doing *Safety Differently*.

In doing *Safety Differently,* the story of the multiple conditions that had to exist for either failure or success to happen became more significant in understanding the work. It is in this thinking the value of understanding normal work moved to the forefront of event learning. We no longer need a failure to investigate work.

Investigating differently

Of all the clear advantages in understanding safety in a different way, is the ability to completely improve our ability to learn from events. Investigations, as we have discussed, traditionally were used to identify deficiencies in workers at multiple levels of the organization. The new approach takes the focus away from finding places where the worker somehow failed the organization and moved this focus towards finding places where the organization and its systems failed the workers.

Some of the highlights of learning differently are listed for your attention. Feel free to compare and contrast these ideas with the way your organization currently does event learning. The differences are exciting. More importantly, these differences allow for a whole new collection of event context information.

The lesson for us is painfully clear, if your organization wants better investigation outcomes then the organization must do better investigations. Here are some different concepts for event learning:

- **Things go wrong all the time in our daily operations.** In most instances, workers detect and correct problems in real-time. Failure happens all the time; all the components for an unwanted outcome live in your organizational system and processes as a part of daily work. An organization can learn from typical work much better than from waiting for an event.

- **Events are the unexpected combination of normal work contexts.** Don't look for some type of special deviation to explain why an event happened. Instead, look at the work as it is done when it does not fail. Learn how this work is done when it does not fail to better understand the conditions present when the work fails.

- **Investigations learn/Corrective actions fix.** There is a huge difference between learning and fixing. Learning always must happen *before* fixing. Too often organizations do investigations to fix problems. Investigating to fix problems will ensure the organization will not learn enough about the work to truly understand what happened. It is much better to see the corrective actions as a product of the learning analysis. Your organization must learn before it can act.

- **Investigations answer the "how" question, not the "why" question.** When an event happens, there is a desperate need to answer the "why" question. Many organizations are so fixated on the "why" question they use a stair-step process of asking the why question many times. Our organization desperately wants to understand "why something bad happened."

There is a caution here, the mysterious "why" question is much less useful to the organization than the very practical and informative "how" question. "How" allows the organization to move beyond individual motivation and to focus more on the complex conditions that had to exist for the failure to happen. Stick with "how."

- **Tell the story of the conditions necessary to have the failure that happened.** Complex systems are made up of many separate parts that are tightly coupled together. Identifying the individual parts of the event, the conditions present for the event to happen helps to illustrate the complex nature of an event. Traditional investigations tend to put preferential treatment on the combination of all the individual parts of an event. This is evident in traditional investigation timelines, highlighting process deviation and root cause analysis.

One of the best motivations for doing *Safety Differently* is the opportunity to change the organization's approach to event learning. Deliberately learning the contextual factors present in an event by changing the actual event learning foundation will help the organization understand an event, and more importantly the event context, in a more effective way. The opportunity to seek the richer question of how the event happened offers the organization a more complete understanding of the event.

Even more effective is the realization that this new event learning technique does not need to be used only to understand a failure. These tools, because they focus on understanding the multiple conditions present in the work environment, also function in helping the organization to better understand typical work. There is no need to wait for an event to learn.

When is the last time your organization used traditional investigation tools to look at normal work?

Discussion questions

1. If you were to ask your own organization why it does investigations, what do you think the answer would be? Should you try to change that?

2. Do you have any examples of 'successful failures' in your own organization that were mostly hailed as a success and that inspired further improvements?

3. Why is thinking in terms of 'root causes' not very helpful?

4. In what sense are the administrative and policy apparatus (and perhaps the politics) surrounding and driving investigations in your organization actually limiting learning and improvement?

5. What is the link between investigating differently and acknowledging the difference between work-as-imagined and work-as-done?

Chapter 4
When there's too much compliance: Declutter your safety bureaucracy

> *"In any bureaucracy, the people devoted to the benefit of the bureaucracy itself always get in control and those dedicated to the goals that the bureaucracy is supposed to accomplish have less and less influence, and sometimes are eliminated entirely."*
>
> - Jerry Pournelle, "The Iron Law of Bureaucracy"

It's easy to write more rules. In a study of hospital wards, colleagues at Macquarie University found that nurses—on average—need to follow 600 policies every day. That's a lot of policies. When they asked nurses if they could recite some of those policies back to them, they got a lot of blank stares. On average, nurses were able to describe between two and three policies. That meant that 597 to 598 of all those policies were lost in the background fog of doing actual work; of taking care of patients daily. It didn't mean that nurses weren't doing what some of these policies specified—they probably were (although they weren't aware of it and didn't need to be). But it *did* mean that there was a whole lot of unnecessary written clutter, inserted into the system by people who were probably as well meaning, as they were ignorant about how work gets done.[22]

Safety and rule clutter has a way of building up around any job, particularly safety-critical jobs. In the US, there has been such a swelling of rules, guidelines, protocols, prescriptions, procedures and policies for administering anesthesia that there are currently some four million documents. Somebody did the math: it takes about 2,000 years to read it all! And then you haven't even trained as a doctor yet.[23]

---

[22] Debono, D. S., Greenfield, D., Travaglia, J. F., Long, J. C., Black, D., Johnson, J., & Braithwaite, J. (2012). Nurses' workarounds in acute healthcare settings: A scoping review. *BMC Health Services Research, 13*, 175-183.

[23] Johnstone, R. E. (2017). Glut of Anesthesia Guidelines a Disservice, Except for Lawyers. *Anesthesiology News, 42*(3), 1-6.

At the same time, the safety yield from every additional operational rule declines as you are getting safer. Remember some of Amalberti's data from the first chapter. If you are an unsafe industry or activity, with chances of one in a thousand ending up with a fatality or serious injury or incident, then writing more operational rules can still increase your safety. But by the time the chances of you badly or fatally injuring someone are down to one per 100,000, they stop having much, if any, effect.[24] The system of writing more rules, Amalberti says, becomes purely additive. It adds more rules to the system, but it offers nothing in return—except more clutter and a bigger compliance apparatus to implement, monitor, audit and control (so of course, *somebody* is winning here). Also, for every new rule added, an old one seldom gets taken out. As said, it's easy to write more rules. It's really difficult to scrap them. Organizational activities and accountabilities abound that all—either regularly or ad hoc—offer many opportunities for the addition of rules. There is typically no similar set of activities and accountabilities for *reducing* the number of rules. And, of course, there can be quite a bit of anxiety around getting rid of rules, which you don't see when rules get added.

---

[24] When your system is as safe as 10^{-5} or one in 100,000, then writing more operational safety rules is not going to change much, other than adding more clutter and making it more difficult to remain compliant. Instead, the data suggests, your safety will benefit from you investing in safety-by-design, in human factors engineering and in a just reporting culture. See: Amalberti, R. (2001). The paradoxes of almost totally safe transportation systems. *Safety Science, 37*(2-3), 109-126.

But safety clutter can be dangerous. It can compound and add risks by making things less transparent. It can muddle the waters by making critical issues less obvious, by creating decoy phenomena that get everybody worried while real trouble is brewing elsewhere. And, as said, it can suck up time and resources without adding anything of value but distracting people from what they should be looking at. The research on disasters shows plenty of examples of this. Just prior to the Space Shuttle Challenger launch decision for example, "bureaucratic accountability undermined the professional accountability of the original technical culture, creating missing signals."[25] Macondo serves as another example. In 2008, two years before the Macondo (or Deepwater Horizon) well blowout, BP warned that it had "too many risk processes" which had become "too complicated and cumbersome to effectively manage."[26]

---

[25] Vaughan, D. (1996). *The Challenger launch decision: Risky technology, culture, and deviance at NASA.* Chicago: University of Chicago Press, p. 363.

[26] Elkind, P., Whitford, D., & Burke, D. (2011, 24 January). BP: 'An accident waiting to happen'. *Fortune, 85*(1), 1-14, p. 9.

You may have experienced unreasonable compliance burdens and a sense of overregulation as well. You're not alone—nor is your organization, your industry, or even your country. So, we'll do a couple of things in this chapter. First, we try to get our heads around 'safety clutter.' What is it exactly? Then we dive into the reasons for increasing clutter. What are the various kitchens in which compliance clutter is cooked up, and what's going on there? Where does all this stuff come from, and why? And finally, of course, we will look at some ways in which you can start safely decluttering.

What is safety clutter?

One of our students was out asking supervisors about which safety practices they liked or disliked. They frequently mentioned problems with 'induction'. On further inquiry, it appeared that contractors were required to complete an online induction process that was intended to take three hours but could take up to six hours for a contractor with low computer literacy. This was only part of the picture, though. As the student explored further, it became clear that the term 'induction' sometimes referred to the online induction, and sometimes to site inductions. Eventually, we realized that there were five separate inductions, each covering roughly the same relevant material, and a variable amount of irrelevant material. Before performing work on a site, a contractor could be required to complete all five inductions – amounting to more than a full day of work. At least on paper, these inductions were required even for a worker who was only spending a few hours on site. To reduce the cost of providing inductions, another organization introduced Computer- Based Training (CBT) inductions. Given the work to be done, not all contractors were entirely literate. One of the contractors became known as the 'super-inductor'. Their employee would sit at seven computer terminals simultaneously, rolling back and forth between them, and making sure every contractor passed the induction. Few of them ever found out what was actually in the induction, but they had passed and were (at least on the record) 'safe' to be on site.[27]

---

[27] Rae, A. J., Weber, D. E., Provan, D. J., & Dekker, S. W. A. (2018). Safety Clutter: The accumulation and persistence of 'safety' work that does not contribute to operational safety. *Policy and practice in health and safety*, 16(2), 194-211.

There's no doubt that your organization also has (supposed) safety activities that are performed with no expectation that they will provide any real safety benefit. Such activities drain time, eat away at resources and deflect attention away from things that could be done to improve the safety of operational work. These activities are an example of safety clutter. Safety clutter doesn't help the reputation of safety or that of safety professionals or human performance experts. They get to be known as the 'fun police,' or as those who get in the way of real workers getting the job done.

So, safety clutter is the accumulation of rules, policies, safety procedures, documents, roles, and activities that are implemented and performed in the name of safety but do not contribute to the safety of operational work. Safety clutter may well distract from those things that could help improve the safety of work.

One popular way to create clutter is simply by duplication. Two or more very similar activities fill the same safety function, but the duplicate activities add no additional safety. We see this a lot in the relationship between contractors and principals. They may both have their processes and procedures for starting or assuring the safety around a particular task. Depending on how responsibilities are managed on a site, it is quite likely that each of these processes needs to be discharged. That way, both the contractor and the principal can fulfill their due diligence obligations (at least in the accountability paper trail up the organizational hierarchy).

Clutter by duplication is not the same as intentional repetition or redundancy. For example, an operation might deliberately have a safety-critical instrument reading or calculation cross-checked by two different people as a form of redundancy. Or it might repeat the activity at set intervals as a form of monitoring. Redundancy and monitoring, used appropriately, can sometimes reduce risk, but only under tightly scripted conditions.[28]

But clutter can take many other forms. Perhaps the most ridiculous clutter is also the most irritating for those who prefer to use common sense, who want to be taken seriously, and want to get work done. This sort of clutter comes from role and rule creep: the gradual spreading of safety rules or symbols that were never intended for the place they end up. But once there, they lose relevance and credibility — even if they can still get enforced. Here are some examples that our colleagues and we have found:

- Signs on stairs instructing workers to 'maintain 3 points of contact,' which were

---

[28] The problem is called the 'fallacy of social redundancy.' You might believe that having two people checking something (a process, a calculation, an instrument reading) introduces the kind of reliability that you get when you put redundancy in an engineered system (where the probability of the whole failing is the product (i.e., multiplication) of the probabilities of the individual parts failing. Multiplying two numbers that are both smaller than one will result in an even smaller probability number). That's not the case if the *people* are supposed to form the redundancy (i.e., the redundancy is social). People make assumptions about each other. They get to know each other. They might skip something, or not look as carefully, because they know the other person will also look and pick up anything untoward. Except the other person can think that too. The result is that the probability of the whole failing may well be larger than either of the two constituent parts (humans) failing. That's why social fallacy is generally a fallacy, unless it's carefully wrapped inside various standardized practices, briefings, callouts and the like.

taken from safety rules for the use of ladders. One organization even instructed 4 points of contact on stairs. It was pointed out to them that movement was then impossible, after which they quickly clarified that the fourth point of contact was intended as 'eye contact;'

- Duplicate labels warning users that a hot tap will issue hot water taken from hazardous area warning labels, or labels on-site toilets that use grey (storm) water for flushing that say 'not for drinking';

- Risk assessments for travel to be done on a seven-page form, independent of whether such travel was to a remote, risk-filled country on another continent or to a neighboring city in the same state.

If a safety group is given too much sway over what happens on the operational front-end, then there is a risk of — what sociologists call — bureaucratic entrepreneurism. People who feel newly empowered can impose rules on others, which at the same time gives them more to do, more authority to do it, and surrounded by an aura of inevitability. They can even claim that what they are doing is both ethical and necessary and that those who disagree are not taking safety seriously.

You can see this in another form of clutter too: over-specification. This is quite a popular way to extend safety clutter. It often connects to recording and accountability requirements, which are intended to demonstrate that certain activities or steps are done.

In one such case, an offshore foreman lamented that his company had just introduced a new procedure for how to clean a sand filter on a pump. The new procedure contained 147 steps, each of which needed to be signed off. He'd been working offshore and cleaning sand filters for close to 40 years, and probably knew what he was doing. But the most interesting part was this: he actually couldn't do the job when following the 147 steps. His 'flow,' based on visual cues, prompts and muscle memory, would disintegrate when he was only a few steps into the process. It was like telling a pianist who is an expert at playing a difficult classical piece by heart that she now needed to go back to the notes and follow each one of them carefully (and sign off each one when it was played). The performance would suffer greatly, and the pianist would probably only get a few measures into the piece before giving up.

Of course, the foreman also wondered about the practicality of having a stack of paper out on the deck, when his (gloved) hands would be on the various parts of the filter and the pump. He didn't even have to mention the fact that the wind often blows hard across the deck and that the weather can generally be wet and crappy. If anybody believed that the 147-step procedure would follow the foreman out on the deck, to be filled out in real-time (as had been the intention of his company), then they must have been dreaming. The clutter was produced by someone who had never been out on an oil rig before. But that someone had the power to determine how work was supposed to happen there and was concerned about fulfilling bureaucratic accountability requirements around safety and compliance.

Overspecification is a form of clutter that fits with a particular trend: that of deprofessionalization. We'll talk about that more below, but you probably know what we mean: a gradual loss of trust and confidence in professionals to take responsibility to do their jobs well, robbing them of a sense of pride, autonomy and achievement.

Where does safety clutter come from?

Here's an eye-opener for you:

> "The largest source of growth in rules and regulations is the private sector. We tend to blame the government for bureaucracy's drag on our productivity, but the dollars locked up by businesses in complying with self-imposed red tape are double those associated with government regulations."[29]

---

[29] Thus said Giam Swiegers, CEO of Deloitte Australia. In Saines, M., Strickland, M., Pieroni, M., Kolding, K., Meacock, J., Nur, N., & Gough, S. (2014). *Get out of your own way: Unleashing productivity.* Sydney, Australia: Deloitte Touche Tohmatsu, p. 1.

So, the government is *not* the problem. On average, three out of every five rules are made up and self-imposed by organizations. Only two of the five rules can be traced back to a regulation or government requirement, this same study found. In some sectors, it's much worse than that. Finance is one of them. Healthcare is another. 85% of its compliance demands are those that it has produced itself, as an industry — related to how it bills, accounts, distributes, responsibilizes, trains and checks.[30] One ICU doctor in Texas told us that she could easily fill each 12-hour shift with 16 hours of paperwork and compliance activities. (We couldn't get the math to work out on that one either, except that we figured that she wouldn't see a single patient during the entire shift.)

---

[30] Carayon, P., & Cassel, C. K. (2019). *Taking action against clinician burnout: A systems approach to professional well being.* Washington, DC: National Academy of Sciences, Engineering, and Medicine.

There is a link with the government. But it probably isn't what you think. Interestingly, we have seen the rise in safety clutter and compliance burdens precisely because of *deregulation*.[31] This may seem counterintuitive but think about it. Since the 1990s, there has been a shift from compliance-based regulation in many industries to risk- or performance-based regulation. Under such a regime, the government no longer comes in regularly to check, with its people, whether you are compliant with every little specification, rule and regulation that it had on the books for you. With the increasing complexity and sophistication of many technologies, the government probably no longer even has the in-house expertise to do that well. Instead, you are more on your own, and now you have to demonstrate to the government that you know your risks and that you have them under control.

---

[31] Dekker, S. W. A. (2021). *Compliance Capitalism: How free markets have led to unfree, overregulated workers.* London: Routledge.

How many organizations and industries have responded to this requirement is the same as what we see in some freshmen students. When asked a question on a test, they will throw *everything* at the professor they've ever learned in the course (never mind word limits). They do this just to make sure that they're sort of compliant with expectations and hope that what's needed to answer the question is buried in there, somewhere. Organizations similarly overcompensate—richly. They're even helped in that by others (e.g., compliance consultants) who are all too happy to sell them stuff they don't need (bloated safety management systems, for instance), which they then offer to maintain on your behalf (for a healthy fee, of course).

This is why deregulation has actually created a sense of overregulation, and how it ironically ends up imposing unreasonable compliance demands. It explains why most of the rules that you have to follow today are made up by your organization, not by the government. Just think about it. The government didn't put that sign up on your stairway that said you needed to 'maintain four points of contact.' Your organization did. Either way, you don't need it, because you probably know since childhood how to walk up and down stairs. The interaction between a retreating government, which may genuinely be trying to get out of the way to make things better and easier, and the response of the private sector can be more complex than that, though. Here is a great example.[32]

---

[32] You can find this example, and many other great ones, in: Dekker, S. W. A. (2021). *Compliance Capitalism: How free markets have led to unfree, overregulated workers.* London: Routledge.

The first substantive policy that Bush signed into law, in March 2001, was a repeal of the Occupational Safety and Health Administration's (OSHA's) ergonomics program standard. The congressional vote that had preceded this was surrounded by an intense campaign by human factors and ergonomics professionals, but it was ultimately unsuccessful. The federal ergonomics standard had to go; the regulator had to pull its head in. The repeal of a federal ergonomics standard wouldn't seem like the thing you'd get excited about. After all, the standard mostly involved paper bureaucracy and the sort of work that doesn't typically kill people or trigger devastating, highly visible accidents. But it became a perfect example of deregulation that ends up causing organizational self-inflicted overregulation.

It became a case where a retreating government – under pressure from free-market proponents – drove the so-called 'responsibilization' of workers who now became tasked with assessing and regulating ergonomic standards by and for themselves, and who had to carry the can if they didn't. It was a case of a politically marketable effort to reign in a putatively overreaching, intrusive government, to stop them from overburdening businesses with seemingly gratuitous paperwork. And it led to businesses imposing seemingly gratuitous paperwork on their workers instead (of course, without them giving up any of their productivity). Duly signed off, all this paperwork could then let businesses off the hook for workplace ergonomic injuries. It was a case where a retreating government made space for a new market in which private insurers and purveyors of occupational safety, and ergonomics consultants, could capitalize on liability fears and then sell products to businesses keen on avoiding trouble and costs associated with injury claims.

What had been the problem that the Occupational Health and Safety Authority (OSHA) was trying to tackle with the ergonomics standard? And what did Bush repeal? Personal computers had only just become the dominant thing on people's desks. OSHA, a division within the US Department of Labor, saw trouble looming. Long hours of computer work would lead to an explosion of musculoskeletal disorders (MSDs), particularly repetitive strain injuries (RSIs) to hands and wrists, spreading to arms and necks and backs and more. Explaining its proposed rulemaking, which OSHA had to submit under the 1995 Paperwork Reduction Act (an indication that the state already knew it created too much compliance paperwork), OSHA argued:

> *These disorders cause persistent and severe pain, lost work time, reduction or loss of the worker's normal functional capacity both in work tasks and in other of life's major activities, loss of productivity, and significant medical expenses. Where preventive action or early medical intervention is not provided, these disorders can result in permanent damage to musculoskeletal tissues, causing such disabilities as the inability to use one's hands to do even the small tasks of daily life (e.g., lifting a child), permanent scarring, and arthritis.*[33]

---

[33] OSHA. (2000). Supporting statement for paperwork reduction act 1995 submissions: Ergonomics Program Standard. Notice of Proposed Rulemaking (Federal register #64). Washington, DC: Occupational Safety and Health Administration, US Department of Labor.

For OSHA to come this far was a victory in itself. A coalition of organized labor, women's groups, and committees on occupational safety and health fought for two decades to secure the ergonomics standard. From ground level, after all, it hadn't been hard to see how RSIs had dramatically increased with the spread of repetitive motion and computer work in both blue-collar and white-collar sectors of the economy. After the 1994 Republican takeover of control of Congress, the Clinton administration had been forced to make numerous concessions to the ergonomics standard, and it was finally signed in the closing days of his presidency. OSHA proposed that MSD-injured employees should be compensated for up to 90 days with both pay and benefits. The standard was going to affect about 102 million workers at some 6 million worksites across the United States and was estimated to cost employers about $4.5 billion per year.

Pulling the government out and letting the market do its work voluntarily was going to change all that. The government was going to get out of the way: on 20 March 2001, Bush signed the repeal of the OSHA rules that had taken effect only a few weeks earlier, four days before he was sworn in. In the doublespeak typical of such occasions, Bush' 20 March signing statement assured his people that:

> *The safety and health of our Nation's workforce is a priority for my Administration. Together we will pursue a comprehensive approach to ergonomics that addresses the concerns surrounding the ergonomics rule repealed today. We will work with Congress, the business community, and our Nation's workers to address the important issues.*[34]

Of course, Congress proceeded to not do much of anything about the 'important issues' because it was now up to the market to address them through voluntary compliance. The business community's 'important issue' (don't cost us any money) became a honeypot for new market actors attracted to selling products that could deal with lingering fears of liability for ergonomic injury. And the Nation's workers got more compliance pressure and less protection. The private sector is keenly set to work to address the Bush administration's concerns about OSHA's standard.

About ten years later one of us was giving a talk about compliance pressure and nonsensical company rules when one of the middle managers volunteered a great example. It was the 'how to sit at your desk checklist' that his company had just adopted. The provider of the checklist was an ergonomics consultancy, and it quickly dawned on the company that they could save on insurance premiums for worker's compensation if they adopted the checklist. He handed us a copy of the checklist after the talk. It was four pages long. Here are some extracts.

<u>*How to sit at your desk*</u>
Workers have to check YES or NO to the following questions (the original working-at-a-desk checklist runs for four pages):

CHAIR
  1. Is the chair easily adjusted from a sitting position?

---

[34] Saunders, T. G. (2001). Bill Files 03/20/2001 [S.J.R. 6]. George W. Bush Presidential Library, FRC ID 778([S.J.R. 6]), p. 33.

2. Is the backrest angle adjusted so that you are sitting upright while keying, and is it exerting a comfortable support on the back?
3. Does the lumbar support of the backrest sit in the small of your back (to find the small of your back, place your hands on your waist and slide your hands around to your spine? The maximum curve of the backrest should contract this area)
4. Are your thighs well-supported by the chair except for a 3-4 finger space (approx.) behind the need (you may need to adjust the backrest of your chair to achieve this)
5. Is there adequate padding on the chair (you should be able to feel the supporting surface underneath the foam padding when sitting on the chair)?
6. If you have a chair mat, is it in good condition?

DESK
1. Is your chair high enough so that your elbows are just above the height of the desk (note: to determine elbow height relax your shoulders and bend your elbows to about 90 degrees)?
2. Are your elbows by your sides and shoulders relaxed?
3. Are your knees at about hip level, i.e., thighs parallel to the floor (may be slightly higher or lower depending on comfort)?
4. Is there adequate legroom beneath your desk?
5. Do you require a footrest?

SCREEN
1. When sitting and looking straight ahead, are you looking at the top one-third of your screen?
2. Is your screen at a comfortable reading distance (i.e., approximately an arm's length away from your seated position)?
3. Can you easily adjust and position your screen?

4. Are all the characters on the display legible and the image stable (i.e., not flickering)?
5. Do light reflections on your screen cause you discomfort (you may need to adjust the angle of your screen)?
6. Do you wear bifocal glasses during computer work?
7. Do you have dual monitors at your workstation?

KEYBOARD

1. Is your keyboard positioned close to the front edge of your desk (approximately 60-70mm from the edge)?
2. Is the keyboard sitting directly in front of your body when in use?
3. Does it sit slightly raised up?
4. If the keyboard is tilted, are your wrists straight, not angled, when typing?
5. Are the keys clean and easy to read?

MOUSE/LAPTOP

1. Are your mouse and mouse pad directly beside the end of the keyboard, on your preferred side?
2. Do you use a laptop computer for extended periods of time at a desk?
3. Is the screen raised so that the top of the screen is at eye level?
4. Do you use an external keyboard and mouse?

DESK LAYOUT

1. Are all the items that you are likely to use often within easy reach?
2. Is there sufficient space for documents and drawings?
3. If most of your work requires typing from source documents, do you require a document holder?

4. *If you use a document holder, is it properly located close to your monitor and adjustable?*
5. *Is your workstation set out to prevent undue twisting of your neck and back?*

The checklist, the manager said to me, took about 20 minutes to fill out, even after you got routinized at it. After filling it out, the worker had to take the completed checklist to his or her Safety Professional who had to sign it and then to the Safety Manager who also had to sign it (these titles are capitalized on the checklist form, we're not making this up). Each completed checklist was kept on record in the worker's personnel file.

The company, in a bid to save money and increase efficiencies on its office staff, then decided to institute hot-desking. This meant that no worker had his or her 'own' desk anymore, but that workstations had to be grabbed in the morning on a first-come, first-serve basis. With each new workstation, however, a new ergonomics self-assessment had to be conducted and a checklist needed to be filled out. The checklist now took 20 minutes out of every workday, or 40 if you were unlucky enough to lose your desk space over a lunch break. There were probably workers who snuck a stack of checklists home with them so that they could pre-fill them for the week or month to come (or have their kids do it just for the heck of it). That way, they could at least get on with their jobs after arriving at yet another random hot desk in the morning.

Remember how proponents of the repeal from the example above had argued that vague government provisions would lead to undue compliance burdens on employers. These vague provisions were now exported, with the help of a private market actor, to the workers. As free agents, as self-regulating beings, they now had to make determinations about what constituted 'slightly raised up,' 'adequate legroom,' 'easily adjusted,' or 'good condition.' These were all pretty vague judgment calls, of course, unless you did ergonomics for a living. The point was never to make workers ergonomically comfortable or safe, the middle manager assured me, even though the checklist was cloaked in exactly that intention.

But if that were the real aim, it would have required some professional help to the workers about what all these things meant, how they should be determined, and what should be done if some of them didn't meet the 'vague' standard. No, the manager said, the point was to save money on insurance premiums and compensation claims. After all, if a worker had ticked the box that assured his or her Safety Professional and then Safety Manager that there was 'no undue twisting of neck and back,' then there was no basis for a claim about the neck- or back pain induced at work.

The example of how to sit at your desk is a great example of deregulation and free markets at work. Here, roughly, is the playbook:

- Get rid of the regulation and get rid of the regulator if you can. Tell the state to stay away.

- Then give everything a price, or, rather, let the markets set a price for everything, including injury.

- Abolish the state's worker compensation scheme and outsource injury compensation to the private insurance market instead.

- Allow the burgeoning of a consultancy market where someone will come up with a 'how-to-sit-at-your-desk-checklist' and sell it to you by sowing fear about what it might cost you if you don't buy it.

- Then responsibilize your workers to do their self-regulatory work by plodding through that checklist every time they go sit at a desk, and implicitly or explicitly warn them of making 'poor choices' when working at their stations.

- Then hold your workers accountable for compliance with your new rules through this arduous four-page long process that will allow you to pass the buck back to the worker when it turns out that they got RSI after all.

This is an instructive example of how free markets lead to safety clutter and to unfree, overregulated (and maybe even poorer and unhealthier) workers. The repeal of the ergonomics standard was a case of less money and less work for the state, of less money and more work for the workers, and of more money and more work for private actors who quickly found their feet in a new market for do-it-yourself-ergonomic standards and assessments. With Bush repealing the federal standard, everything changed. And yet very little did, except who now had to put up with increased safety clutter and paperwork, and who lost, and who won.

Freedom in a frame

Freedom-in-a-frame means that you give your people a framework within which to work (framed by rules or boundaries that you jointly develop and agree on), but within which you give them the freedom and discretion to do their work in the way they see fit. This is a kind of discretionary space, a space that can be filled only by an individual human. This is a final space in which the organization does leave people freedom of choice (to use this tool or not, to launch or not, to go to open surgery or not, to fire or not, to continue an approach or not). It is a space filled with ambiguity, uncertainty and moral choices. Organizations, and however many frames they create, can never substitute the responsibility borne by workers within that discretionary space. Workers would not even want their responsibility to be taken away by systems and processes and frames. The freedom (and the responsibility and accountability it comes with) that is left for them is what makes them and their work human, meaningful, a source of pride.

Freedom in a frame acknowledges and deploys the kind of professional autonomy and trust that allows people to know the boundaries of their roles and authority, yet encourages self-sufficiency, adaptive capacity, interpretive discretion and local innovation. Some examples exist in the private sector that offer an antidote to bureaucratic clutter. Younger companies like Netflix, for instance, may allow people the autonomy to make up their minds about what is the right thing to do in many instances. Their *entire* expense reimbursement policy, for instance, might read 'do right by Netflix.' These are super-refreshing examples (which, even at Netflix, don't fully extend to their safety organization yet...). Unfortunately, many other private-sector workers can find themselves enmeshed in a centrally controlled and micromanaged bureaucracy. They are sometimes no longer trusted to govern themselves as professionals under that sort of we're-in-this-together cooperative ethic.

But perhaps the most surprising examples come from the government, and how it actually can empower its workers to be self-sufficient, self-directed, autonomous and free to choose what the right thing is to do. Why might you find more of this in government jobs? Reasons that have been mentioned include the slightly looser focus on results and money (and thus on accounting and accountability), as well as the typically less precarious employment relations.[35] Kaufman's book The Forest Ranger from 1960 describes how 792 semi-autonomous forest rangers — each with jurisdiction over vast swaths of federal land — were able to make reasonably consistent decisions about grazing rights, timber harvest, fire protection, and scores of other necessary choices regarding the use of public resources. Kaufman captures the public culture in which:

- Rangers internalized certain common professional values;
- Rangers shared a sense of joy at taking, and being given, responsibility;
- Rangers had a 'neutral competency' themselves, allowing them to master their work and their areas of responsibility;
- There was only 'soft' and distant oversight by their employing agency;
- A rotation system kept the rangers from going entirely native or being captured by local interests in their work areas;

---

[35] Lorenz, C. (2012). If You're So Smart, Why Are You under Surveillance? Universities, Neoliberalism, and New Public Management. *Critical Inquiry, 38*(3), 599-629.

- The rotation system also ensured the sharing and distribution of novel solutions across different jurisdictions over time.[36]

There is a fascinating and little-known historical footnote to this. To achieve these results, the US Forest Service had been inspired by *Prussian* methods of administration. Of course, the Prussians are commonly (or stereotypically) seen as perhaps the most rigorous and inflexible of Germans. But that's true only on the surface. In his instructors to commanders, Field Marshall von Moltke wrote in 1869:

- Don't order more than necessary and avoid planning beyond the situation you can foresee;

- Subordinates are justified in modifying or even changing the task assigned, as long as it supports the higher commander's intent (he called this *Auftragstaktik*, or 'Assignment tactics')

- Look for those with *Verantwortungsfreudligkeit*, who have willingness and a joy at taking responsibility for others and for the work they need to jointly accomplish. They like taking ownership and take pride in doing so.

---

[36] The advantages of such rotations were 'rediscovered' by high-reliability organization theorists more than two decades later in a study of sailors employed by the US Navy, another huge government bureaucracy.

Several of the things that the Forest Service relied on came directly from this Prussian playbook. Recruit those who have this sense of *Verantwortungsfreudkligkeit*. Offer them freedom in a frame. Instill agency-inspired values and beliefs in those who joined it—which had existed before but been formalized as a mode of governance by the Prussians.

This should be instructive for us. Deregulated industries don't guarantee a life free from the compulsion of rules or the presence of bureaucratic control. The opposite appears to be true: this has consistently led to intensive managerial control practices and more bureaucracy. A good contrast to think about is that between Theory X and Theory Y of work (and workers)—a distillation of the ideas above by Doug McGregor back in 1960. Theory X managers tend to take a pessimistic view of their workers. They assume that they are naturally unmotivated and that they dislike work. So, workers need to be prompted, rewarded, cajoled, monitored or punished the whole time to make sure that they complete their tasks.

Theory X assumes that workers:

- Hate their work
- Avoid responsibility and need constant direction
- Have to be controlled, forced and threatened to deliver work
- Need to be supervised at every step
- Have no incentive to work. They have no ambition and need to be externally motivated to achieve goals.

Organizations with a Theory X approach typically have several layers of managers and supervisors who oversee and direct workers. There is plenty of surveillance, authority doesn't get delegated. Control remains firmly centralized. Managers are more authoritarian and actively intervene, ostensibly to get things done. Theory X requires all frames and offers no freedom.

McGregor's Theory Y, in contrast, has a more upbeat view of people. It tends toward a more decentralized, participative style of management. It both builds and relies on trust and collaboration to get things done and doesn't drive systems of surveillance and control to check that they indeed are. Instead, people have greater responsibility, and managers encourage them to develop skills and suggest improvements.

Theory Y assumes that:

- Most people like their work
- There is such a thing as intrinsic motivation
- People's needs and organizational needs can overlap
- Most people like to take responsibility, initiative and ownership if given the opportunity
- Most people are capable of solving problems creatively and imaginatively
- Talent gets underutilized a whole lot.

Theories of motivation keep telling us about the three pillars for allowing people to be intrinsically motivated to do the right thing.[37] They are:

- Autonomy—the ability to control and direct your work—what, when and with whom
- Mastery—the ability to develop your knowledge and skills and expertise, getting better at what you do
- Purpose—the answer to 'why': the sense that you're part of something larger than you are accomplishing together with other people.

When you look at this sort of research, you realize that a lot of what you need to know about safety clutter is not about safety. It is about work, and people, and about what drives them (and what puts them off). This also means that we have good levers for changing the march of safety clutter. Let's turn to those now.

How to reduce your safety clutter

It isn't very easy to reverse a 30-year worldwide trend toward deregulation and self-regulation. This is precisely what has contributed to so much internal safety clutter that you have to deal with now. There's a lot of internal processes and politics that now drive the cluttering and clogging of your organization from the inside out.

---

[37] Some of the original research is in Deci, E. L., Ryan, R. M., & Koestner, R. (1999). A meta-analytic review of experiments examining the effects of extrinsic rewards on intrinsic motivation. *Psychological Bulletin, 125*(6), 659-672, and it was popularized recently by Pink, D. H. (2009). *Drive: The surprising truth about what motivates us*. New York: Riverhead Books.

As we said above, a lot of clutter is the result of knee-jerk responses, driven by the social, reputational and psychological need to take action in response to unplanned and unwanted events and circumstances. This is particularly true in cases that relate to the safety of workers. Managers often have a strong desire to feel (or regain) a sense of control, and they in turn may have to demonstrate that they live up to their responsibilities and accountabilities. This easily leads to the introduction of additional safety work into the organization, with no benefit for the safety of operational work. Safety clutter is driven by this focus on quickly (at least optically) resolving moments of crisis and psychological uncertainty. It isn't concerned so much with the long-term effectiveness of solutions, and there is seldom any systemic follow-up to see whether the 'solutions' are creating more problems than they solved.

The kind of clutter that is driven by bureaucratic entrepreneurism — where people concerned with the 'work of safety,' rather than 'the safety of work' get or take the opportunity to colonize an area of practice that was previously untouched by them — doesn't necessarily follow an incident. It is enough to have a dose of *'what if?'* thinking to trigger an uncritical, cluttering safety intervention. 'What if there was an accident?' 'What if someone tripped?' It is not the probability, but the potential severity of the consequences (not so much for the person involved in the incident, but rather for the liability of those employing or contracting them) that tends to drive this. Copying safety interventions from other organizations plays a role here too.

There are several ways to push back on the kinds of knee-jerk responses and bureaucratic entrepreneurism that lead to safety clutter. Here are empowering insights that you can use as a starting point:

- Most of your safety clutter is self-imposed. Your organization wrote it. That means that your organization has the power to change it.

- A lot of safety clutter is the result of knee-jerk reactions to (badly investigated) incidents (see Chapter 3 about how you can do this better and prevent the writing of yet another rule in response to the latest event).

- Resolve that for each new rule you put in, you take at least one (or better still, two or three) out.

- More internal rules do not equal better legal protection.

- The more self-imposed rules you have, the more likely you will be found out of compliance. The more rules you have, in other words, the easier you may get into trouble.

- You can start decluttering by asking your people *'what's the stupidest thing we're asking you to comply with to work here today?'* You'll learn a lot if you're open to the answers. Engaging with those who do the work, and with how they actually get work done, is key to decluttering.

- If you want to take a serious stab at decluttering, make sure you've only got operational people in the room. No safety people or lawyers. They can have their say (if at all) later.

- You can safely declutter by making sure that only rules directly traceable to a regulation, law or government requirement are on your books.

- You can safely declutter by micro-experimenting (see Chapter 7).

Discussion questions

1. Are there any rules or policies in your organization that you are supposed to follow and that you wouldn't even have known about if it weren't for some occurrence?

2. Do you consider your organization 'cluttered' with rules, policies and procedures? Where do you think it all comes from? And to what extent do safety requirements contribute to all this clutter?

3. Why can safety clutter be dangerous? Is your organization aware of these dangers?

4. How is it possible that government deregulation has caused *greater* safety clutter inside your organization?

5. How would you introduce the idea of 'Freedom in a Frame' into your own organization? What would be the frame and what would be the freedom?

Chapter 5
When your safety people are dejected: Empower them differently

Ding...

When you get on a commercial airline the flight attendant gives you a preflight briefing. They tell you all the important things you should know about flying on a plane. You have probably seen this briefing many times. When the flight attendant gets to the oxygen masks, the attendant always informs the passengers that "if you are flying with a child, please put your mask on before you assist your child." The lesson here is that you must first ensure your stability before you can assure stability for the people around you. This is also true for the transition you are making within your organization.

This book chapter is symbolically about putting your mask on before you assist others in putting on their masks. Although we will not be putting on emergency oxygen (or we certainly hope we won't), we are going to introduce the idea that your safety team will better serve your organization in successfully moving towards seeing *Safety Differently* if you ensure you take care of the safety people in your organization before you diffuse these ideas out to the rest of your organization.

The fun police

Safety people are the ones who inflict bureaucracy and compliance and restrictions on others. That is, at least, a popular belief. They are the ones who are behind the rules and surveillance — if not the creators of it, then at least the purveyors of it — on behalf of the organization. This belief gives everybody else someone to blame and poke fun at. It's the 'safety police.' They are to blame! And safety police:

- thinks they're better than everyone else, but
- doesn't understand what real work is;
- takes away the fun from being at the frontline;
- has lots of petty rules to dish out and no clue;
- comes and tries to record and report stuff that is easily made up, hidden or manipulated.

As said, this is a popular belief. And there's probably some truth to it. Those involved with occupational health and safety, those who do human performance work, they spoil it for the real workers.

But what if safety people themselves are also the recipients of compliance demands and invasive surveillance? What if they feel disempowered, overruled, a cog in a larger system, without a good sense of how they're actually contributing to a greater good?

We were talking to a lecture hall full of safety professionals. As the presentation wound its way to what it does to workers when they are put under surveillance and multiple compliance demands, one in the audience spoke up. "You are describing us!" she said. "This is exactly how we feel!" She went on to explain the multitude of seemingly irrelevant reporting and recording requirements she and her colleagues had to abide by every month. She talked about being compelled into rolling out a policy or campaign they knew wasn't going to have any effect (and that would hurt their credibility and standing even further). But most, she talked about being isolated, secluded, and away from the places where actual safety-critical work was going on. About how she didn't get a chance to go out much to learn about work-as-done because of the stacks of bureaucratic work she had to complete every day. About how she had stopped believing that much of those bureaucratic accountability requirements had anything to do with the safety of work on the frontlines. About how powerless she felt in her ability to change any of it.

When philosopher Hannah Arendt was writing up her observations on totalitarianism in 1967,[38] she may not have known that her reflections would ring true to safety professionals half a century later. Totalitarianism is a system of governance in which all decision-making is centralized with a small team of people at the top. Decisions and orders get imposed on others without giving them much of a chance for input, dissent, or protest. Others are just expected to comply. Surveillance and control are rife. Others are seldom asked to contribute with their opinion, experience or knowledge.

What does this kind of governance, this sort of regime, do to people? Arendt wondered. She found three main characteristics of people living under totalitarianism:

- **Optic compliance**. People do as if they care about the rules. They will comply—or they make their behavior 'look' like they are complying—when they know someone is watching; when they know they are under surveillance. Otherwise they'll just do what they need to do to get on with things. This optic compliance, creating the impression for others that the rules are fine, workable, unproblematic and adhered to.
- **Resignation**. People get resigned when the become learned helpless; when they have started to realize that there's nothing they can do to change the situation they're in. They cannot influence the tasks they're assigned to accomplish; they can't stop nonsensical rules

---

[38] Arendt, H. (1967). *The origins of totalitarianism (Third edition)*. London: George Allen & Unwin Ltd.

coming down the pike for them to implement or follow. They conclude that whatever they do, it's going to be the same anyway.
- **Cynicism**. People become cynical when they stop believing that any of the actions or rules made by others will make any difference, or that they are truly for their benefit. They've been fed so much nonsense or been given so many broken promises, that they wonder whether any of it can be trusted anymore. Intriguingly, Arendt found that people under totalitarianism simultaneously believe everything and believe nothing. One the one hand, they *have* to believe everything, just to keep a glimmer of hope alive among their resigned, optic compliance. But at the same time, weary and jaundiced as they've become, they've learned to no longer believe anything. Cynicism sits at the heart of the paradox.

That safety people might feel resigned and cynical, and sense that they have few other options than to be optically compliant, is an important realization. Because is that really what we had in mind for them? Is that what we want them to be, and do?

A traditional safety role

The compliance, resignation and cynicism that safety people might feel has a lot to do with the role we've carved out for them (perhaps unintentionally) in almost all our organizations. Together with other researchers, we've dug deeply into what this role boils down to, and why. And, of course, we've examined what the alternatives could be. What does an innovated safety role, or safety innovation role, look like?[39] Before we go there, let's have a look at how current safety roles may disempower and disenchant some of the people who do those roles for a living. And what that says about us as organizations, as workers, employers and other stakeholders in the creation of safety.

The traditional role of safety is to help stop everything that can go wrong, from going wrong. You will remember that from the first chapter. This means that:

- Safety management involves a strong focus on barriers, restrictions, standardization and compliance.
- Incidents, accidents and near misses are believed to be the result of workers ignoring those barriers. It's because workers bust the restrictions, because they're being non-compliant.
- The way to govern safety, then, is to centralize it. Don't allow workers to do their own thing, don't permit them to improvise, don't let them

---

[39] You can find the results of this research here: Provan, D. J., Woods, D. D., Dekker, S. W. A., & Rae, A. J. (2020). Safety II professionals: How resilience engineering can transform safety practice. *Safety Science, 195,* 1067-1080.

innovate without checking with you first (and you'll probably say 'no' or escalate the request up the ladder). Because anything else would be risky.
- You have to keep workers on the straight-and-narrow. You need to restrict the bandwidth of what you want them to do; and of what you allow them to do.

A lot of effort of safety management goes into finding, recording and reporting deviations from prescribed work of any kind, and then eliminating those deviations. Safe work comes from preventing unsafe variation. Safety is achieved by reducing the likelihood — through whatever means — of deviations from safe work practices, and to contain the consequences of deviations on the off-chance that they do occur.

So what do we ask safety people to do, based on this image of (safe) work? Here's a bit of a list:

- Checking compliance with policy and procedures
- Workplace risk assessments
- Hazard analysis
- Develop or inform company policies
- Conduct safety campaigns
- Write procedures
- Give instructions
- Investigate injuries and incidents and accidents
- Physical inspections
- Audits of workplace behavior
- Record, report and tally deviances

There is a bunch of research into safety management practices and the kinds of activities safety people traditionally get to do. But would you believe that there is actually no compelling empirical evidence that safety people improve the safety outcomes of their organizations by doing any of those things in the list?[40] That in itself is pretty depressing and might lead to cynicism and resignation, of course.

Let's unpack some of the typical work-of-safety activities. Because how is it that these things might lead to a sense of disenchantment and disempowerment for safety people? We can briefly look at the surveillance of frontline work (if by distant, retrospective means) the analysis of hazards, the implementation of controls, the monitoring of compliance, campaigns to standardize a safety culture which prioritizes safety and the delegation of authorities so that safety professionals and line managers decide how work is going to be done safely in any particular area. You can see these in table 6.1.[41]

Work of safety	Official justification	Reason for disenchantment
Surveillance of work	Identify the deviations that lead to unsafe	Surveillance only provides distant, fragmented view of

---

[40] Provan, D. J., Dekker, S. W. A., & Rae, A. J. (2017). Bureaucracy, influence and beliefs: A literature review of the factors shaping the role of a safety professional. *Safety Science, 98*, 98-112.

[41] Partially from: Provan, D. J., Woods, D. D., Dekker, S. W. A., & Rae, A. J. (2020). Safety II professionals: How resilience engineering can transform safety practice. *Safety Science, 195*, 1067-1080, p. 1068.

	outcomes	work
Hazard and risk analysis	Analyze the factors and permutations of failures that can lead to unsafe outcomes	Manipulation of ratings to satisfy a-priori demands or constraints
Implement controls	Put in more barriers or other controls to manage hazards	Workers may see controls as nanny-ish and obstructive
Monitor compliance	Control worker behavior through more surveillance, audits, controls and policies	Workers will do things their own way when you're not watching
Delegate authorities	Safety decisions to be made by line managers and safety people	Line managers get listened to better than safety people
Wage safety culture campaigns	Standardize values, attitudes and beliefs with slogans and posters, (supposedly) prioritize safety over all else	The organization has other priorities than safety, despite what it says, otherwise it wouldn't exist
Record and report deviations	Tallies of deviances for different stakeholders	Abstracted numbers pushed up the organizational hierarchy to fulfill bureaucratic accountability obligations and manage liability

Table 1: some typical traditional safety interventions to be undertaken by safety people in an organization that believes in centralized control over the safety of work

Hazard and risk analyses are a great example. They combine our understanding (or, rather, guesses) of probabilities and consequences. The results can be passed up to the organization, for them to decide on the kinds of priorities and resources that are made available for activities and barriers to reduce those risks. Not surprisingly, a hazard or risk analysis often begins with the outcome you want from the organization (or that the organization wants from *you*). How much in the way of resources, restrictions and barriers do we want (or can we put up with) for this particular (set of) tasks? On the basis of the answer to that question, a particular rating then gets assigned to that hazard or risk.

Sometimes a particular rating gets chosen because the people who conduct the analysis already know the organization is not going to give more resources to deal with it, or because they want to help the organization avoid having to make such resourcing commitments. It is understandable that a kind of cynicism can easily slip into this activity. It's just an example, but it goes for other activities of safety people as well. This leads to safety work that can be seen as reactive, distant, fragmented and defensive:

- **Reactive**: Because of the inevitable gap between work as imagined and work as done, there is a constant need for reactive activities to 'correct' work as actually done. Safety people have to explain incidents;

others expect them to explain them in terms of non-compliance and deviances. They all react by reminding workers of the barriers and procedures already in place, or by inventing new ones to add to the compliance burden.

- **Distant**: Safety people become wrapped up in the 'work of safety,' or all the safety management activities that are performed at a distance and separate from the core functioning of workers at the frontline. That means that there's no guiding principle for all that work of safety coming from how work is actually done (and what is required to make *that* work safe).

- **Fragmented**: The work of safety gets driven by a hodgepodge of legal, organizational and other compliance requirements, reactions to incidents or other bad news, or the inspired thought of a leader who wants another poster campaign because her or his peers have one as well. Initiative-fatigue is a common condition, and of course also contributes to cynicism and resignation.

- **Defensive**: All the work of safety becomes so disconnected from the safety of actual frontline work that it begins to resemble a bulwark against risks and threats that don't even come from the frontline. Rather, a lot of the work of safety (ticking boxes, double-checking, documenting) is about managing another threat: that of legal or other liabilities. These will not affect the workers, but those higher up in the organization. The work of safety is a defensive mechanism to help them stay clear of trouble.

As you may already have picked up in chapter 2, both frontline workers *and* the organization need to engage in various things so that they can adapt around this sort of centralized work-of-safety. In part, it's about keeping up appearances, about making it look as if everybody is in agreement about the way safety is done.

For workers (and this may well include safety people themselves!), ways to adapt around centralized safety control include:

- **Covert work systems**. Work-as-done (the kinds of things that need to be done to really make operations happen) gets hidden from view when the work is subjected to formal scrutiny (audits, inspections, management visits). During those moments of intense surveillance, very little real work is actually going on, and will resume when surveillance is gone. This is, literally, the optic compliance we talked about above.

- **Role retreat**. If initiative and innovation are discouraged, one response is to stick strictly to the requirements and specifications of one's role. People refuse going the extra mile, and will be less willing to collaborate across roles or team boundaries.

- **Renaming and manipulation**. If incidents or injuries give rise to bureaucratic overreaction by the organization, the strategy is to not have them. This is accomplished by calling incidents or injuries something else, or finding other ways to not have evidence of them show up. Interestingly, there are few limits to the creativity that people show here. If only such creativity to be channeled into more productive safety uses...

The organization, however, also needs to adapt around the consequences of centralized safety control. Here are some of the ways in which it does so (sometimes unwittingly):

- **Remain ignorant of work-as-done**. The fluency and smoothness with which work is done efficiently and safely (even if it's not done as imagined) is the result of workers applying and combining expertise and experience. They iron out inconsistencies, contradictions, goal conflicts, resource limitations, tools and procedures that aren't fit for the task, and more. Remaining ignorant of the deep cognitive and collaborative commitments that workers make to 'make work work,' is a safe strategy for those wanting to uphold the relevance of centralized safety control.

- **Discounting**. Problems and issues with frontline work that fall outside of 'work-as-imagined' are discounted or rationalized away so that they once again align with existing plans, production goals and models of risk. Workers are told to 'try harder,' or 'care more.' Because the plan is perfect, the organization immaculate. People (workers) have to stop being a problem that gets in the way of the smooth execution of work-as-imagined.

Safety, in an organization that believes in centralized control over the safety of work, becomes more of a bureaucratic *accountability to* people up the hierarchy. They need to get the numbers that tell them that everything is under control. They need to be shown that all is in the green. Safety, as a result, is no longer so much a keenly interested ethical *responsibility for* people down the hierarchy. Of course it is, as leaders (and many safety people) will claim. But if it was, then why do we put stickers on bathroom mirrors? You know, the stickers that say:

You are looking at the person responsible for your safety

If people are just responsible for their own safety, then what—indeed—is the role of the safety professional? Or, for that matter, what is the obligation that's left for the organization that employs or contracts the person who is looking in the mirror and sees that sticker? Well, in a traditional safety universe, their obligation is to try to make it impossible for workers to do unsafe things or end up in unsafe situations. Work to plan, work to role, work to rule. That's what workers should be doing. Safety professionals encourage and pursue this by trying to foresee, predict and foreclose the kinds of things that shouldn't happen. There's nothing wrong with trying to live up to this obligation—except that there is.

You've already read about it in chapter 2. Work as imagined is *not* the same as work as done. We might think we know how work gets done, and we write rules and procedures for it that way, and we devise barriers to fit around our image of that work. We believe that the plan for safe work is immaculate and complete. If only workers stuck with that plan, all would be good. But except for the simplest, most linear, closed, straightforward, finite tasks, it is impossible to *have* a perfect plan—to foresee and predict and foreclose exactly everything that needs to happen to make things go well, and foresee *all* the ways in which things could go wrong in the real world. That idea is based on a conception of the universe that just doesn't apply to the situations in which most people live and work. This is why it's critical to think about innovating the role of your safety people. Because if they're doing what you've been reading above, then you've got them working in a world that is not the world in which your workers work.

If you put your safety people in a job where they can mostly be reactive, distant, fragmented and defensive, you might easily end up in a downward spiral. More safety problems are identified from a distance (and probably misunderstood as deviations of *some* type, always by *other* people who should know better and try harder to comply). These problems are responded to, likely with additional compliance demands. Fragmented, haphazard, ill-coordinated 'solutions' are rolled out and implemented with no connection to work as actually done (except to make that work even harder). Pressure on workers to conform (or develop more optic compliance) increases. Workers have to develop additional adaptations to work around the new constraints, surveillance and expectations, which creates an even greater distance between work-as-done and work-as-imagined.

The consequences for safety management, and for how safety people might feel about themselves, are almost all negative. You probably know them well: blame culture, inappropriate resource allocation, increased goal conflicts, mismatches between making people responsible but without the resources or sufficient authority to live up to that responsibility; non-value-adding safety clutter, stale models of risk and operations, adversarial relationships, lack of systemic or coordinated interventions, a single focus on worker compliance, ever more investments in bureaucratic accountabilities to protect the organization and its leaders, and manipulated safety reporting metrics.

No wonder your safety people might feel disempowered, cynical, and resigned.

But it doesn't have to be that way. There is, as you might have noted, a strong connection between how your organization sees work and workers, and the role safety people end up having. Let's see how that might be done differently; how you might empower your safety people differently.

Focus on the safety of work, not the work of safety[42]

Most safety people run much less risk of becoming dejected if they are allowed to engage with the safety of work—instead of just the work of safety. The work of safety, as we have discussed above, consists of activities that supposedly have the primary purpose of managing safety. But in reality, the work of safety is a form of organizational, or institutional work that has little to do with the safety of work. The work of safety, in contrast, is necessary to persuade or placate stakeholders. The organization is worthy of its license to operate, because it's got safety under control.

---

[42] David Provan and Drew Rae coined the phrase 'work of safety vs. safety of work.' It is a very apt way to contrast the two approaches to safety management. You can find more here: Rae, A. J., & Provan, D. J. (2019). Safety work versus the safety of work. *Safety Science, 111*, 119-127.

If you look at it really crudely, then the work of safety is a kind of 'PR' exercise, an investment in public (and other) relations, a way to make the organization look good and continue with the blessing of others (including regulators, shareholders, the stock market, the surrounding community) to operate. You probably remember the 'looking good index' from chapter 1. It's no wonder that the work of safety involves so much obsession around this LGI (or, in reality, the LTI and other similar numbers).

That doesn't mean that the work of safety is irrelevant: it has an important role to play, just like any public relations or liability-management activity that allows your organization to keep operating. But it's probably honest to acknowledge the extent to your safety work is exactly that. As an example, one safety professional told us that SMS doesn't stand for Safety Management System, but for Safety *Marketing* System. Because that is what the system does: it markets your safety to the regulator (and other stakeholders). It presents a picture to them that you know what you're doing: that you know your risks and that you've got it all under control. That way the organization can get on with its core business. The work of safety is primarily about persuading all those *other* people; convincing them that you're good to keep going. It's about how you look in the eyes of those stakeholders.

The work of safety, however, is distinct from the safety of work. Research keeps showing that the safety of work gets created, mostly, by those who do the work.[43] Given this, what are some of the things that safety people could do to support this to happen, and make it even better? Have a look at table 6.2. and then we'll talk about it some.

Safety of work	How to do this	Why to do this
Learn about everyday work-as-done	Engage with workers and gain their trust to understand how stuff actually gets done	Discover how safety is created every day by work-as-done Learn about obstacles and difficulties that get in the way of getting stuff done
Support and improve work-as-done	Understand local practices and help workers with how to adapt better and safer	Safety interventions won't have staying power if they don't take work-as-done seriously
Find and try to reduce goal conflicts	Ask about and identify places where workers need to do multiple things simultaneously that (may) actually conflict.	Goal conflicts are at the heart of deviances and drift into failure. Without understanding them, there's neither any hope

---

[43] Woods, D. D., Dekker, S. W. A., Cook, R. I., Johannesen, L. J., & Sarter, N. B. (2010). *Behind human error*. Aldershot, UK: Ashgate Publishing Co.

	Help convince others to re-allocate operational resources to alleviate these goal conflicts.	of being taken seriously by workers, nor of doing much that helps improve the safety of work.
Facilitate information flows and coordinate actions	Create mechanisms to get information where it needs to be (even it it's not welcome there). Coordinate actions across team boundaries to prevent fragmentation of safety initiatives.	You have to get information to those who can make decisions about resources. You may need to prepare them to receive 'bad' news (i.e. that work-as-imagined is not the same as work-as-done) and that there are other ways to support safe working than telling workers to be compliant.
Generate future operational scenarios	Try to sketch possible future scenarios that might come with operational or technological changes.	The world is not static. Safety risks change as work changes. Without anybody looking out for them, the organization may unwittingly embrace risky operational changes or descend into techno-optimism.
Help leaders and others	Make trade-off decisions visible	The organization has other priorities

make sacrifice judgments	for organizational leaders and others, so that they know that there's no free lunch.	than safety, despite what it says, otherwise it wouldn't exist. Economic and production pressures almost always interact with safety. Finding ways to make these interactions visible can support leaders and others in their decisions.
Facilitate learning	Keep the model(s) of risk in an organization up-to-date. Find sources of blame. Hunt down anything that puts downward pressure on people's openness and honesty (including an organization's 'Zero Harm' policy or similar).	Models of risk tend to go stale over time. What may cause incidents today can be very different from before the introduction of a particular technology or operational change. Without trust and confidence that people are in this together, there's no basis for learning and improvement of any of this.

Table 6.2.: the kinds of things safety people can do to support the safety of actual frontline work, rather than just performing the work of safety on behalf of their organization.

- You will recall from chapter 2 that there are really cool ways to learn about work-as-done. Most workers are excited about the opportunity to talk about their work—if they know that you're not about to judge them or hold them against some compliance framework. If you are genuinely interested, they'll notice, and you can win the trust necessary to learn about work-as-done. You get to understand the things that workers have to adapt around, the procedures and tools that don't work, the resources that aren't sufficient, the policies that are irrelevant, stale or out-of-date.

The interesting thing is that a safety professional brings a particular lens to these conversations (yes, a 'safety lens') and probably also some knowledge about the wider organizational goals and constraints that may have eluded those who have their nose close to the grindstone on the frontline somewhere. That means that safety people can combine a range of perspectives to come up with novel insights, with richly informed ways of thinking about work and the organization that makes it (im-)possible. It's a vital role that can help 'unfreeze' the organization and its leaders, and show some pathways to start moving along to reconcile production and safety demands. That, of course, can involve getting different teams together (e.g. technical and operational), and getting them to talk about the obstacles and crunches that show up on the frontline. They may otherwise not know about it, and they are probably both necessary to come to a solution.

Safety people can help organizations sense early signs of trouble. All systems operate under (somewhat) degraded conditions all the time (because there's no organization where *everything* is consistently working perfectly *all* the time!). Sometimes the organization is quite aware of such degradations, but it can also have become inured against the more chronic ones. If there are increases in uncertainties (for example: changes in technology, or new operational demands or conditions like a huge new order or different supplier), then it's likely that safety risks will change as well and possibly not (just) for the better. The possibility to create *risk foresight* is a unique contribution that safety people can make. That is much broader (and possibly radically different from) doing more traditional hazard or risk assessments, because the really interesting risks—the escalating, cascading ones—come from the interdependencies and interactions between all kinds of factors. Risk and hazard analyses traditionally don't have the capability to model those.

With that sort of operational intelligence supplied to others, safety people can be key in discussions about sacrificing production goals (even if temporarily) in order to sort out other issues. Some work teams may be told to hold off, or step back from a particular task. Others may need to receive additional unbudgeted resources to preserve their safety margins given the pressures of the new conditions they are working in. Sacrifice judgments like these shouldn't be seen as failures—failures of planning or compliance—but as successes. And they're worth celebrating. Because they show that the organization genuinely embraces safety as its priority, rather than just proclaiming that on a poster somewhere.

A main goal of facilitating learning is to keep the organization aware of the model(s) of risk it has about its own operations. Instead of waiting for some incident or accident to show the limits of the organization's understanding of it's own safety and risk profile, safety people can help by making visible how operational successes are routinely created. What does it take to make things go well? What capacities are required, in teams, in people, in processes, that routinely creates successful outcomes? It is crucial to understand this, because in the creation of these successes also lie the potential seeds of failure, fatality and destruction.

The reason for that is that operational, organizational success can *only* come from a finely balanced set of trade-offs and sacrifices that people throughout the organization make every day. For example:

- You can't do everything by the book and still get work done in time. This is why we have work-to-rule actions or strikes. Follow all the rules for a change, and everything comes to a grinding halt. The point is not that full compliance is impossible (though it generally is); the point is to know what matters and what doesn't matter in a particular setting.

- You can't keep doing work super-cheaply and still do it safely in the long run. Tools will start breaking, parts won't work.

- You can't run back-to-back shifts and then add some overtime just to meet production demands and think that that doesn't increase risk somewhere along the line.

These trade-offs are not in themselves risky (because things mostly go well). But being aware of them is critical: after all, if something changes or persists for a long time, then your organization may well be skirting closer to the edge of that incident or accident it has been trying to steer clear from all along. The prediction of that incident doesn't lie in meaningless safety metrics. Instead, the prediction of that incident lies in everything you have to do to normally create success. Learn about *that*, and you'll learn about how you might fail.

The face of safety differently

As you might have picked up from this chapter by now, the difference in the way your organization is going to do safety will require your safety staff to change some of the everyday requirements and expectations that have traditionally been demanded from the workers. Many of your organization's safety systems, management systems, and risk identification systems will remain the same, or at least similar to what they've been. What will change is the way you define safety and the way leadership thinks about safety – safety is not just the absence of harm; safety is the presence of operational capacity. That difference may feel like a new flavor of the month, but in reality, this is much more of a shift in how we manage *Safety Differently*.

The safety professionals are the face of new safety. They will not only ensure the organization begins doing *Safety Differently*, but also, they will translate, coach, counsel, and guide the organization at all levels toward a new way of thinking. Ensuring the success of your safety professionals will also ensure the success of the change you want to make in your safety and reliability program. Think of your organization's safety professionals as the primary agents of change – every part of this transition will start with this group. Anything you can do to ensure this group is prepared and supported will help ensure your program will succeed.

We have noticed sometimes the group that has the hardest time thinking about *Safety Differently* in an organization is the safety professionals of the same organization. This group has much invested in the traditional approach to safety; the safety team knows what is expected of them. The safety people understand the systems and processes used to manage safety in your organization. This team has spent years building the current safety program, so of course, there is much at risk if things begin to change. Having pride and a sense of ownership of your organization's current safety program seems completely reasonable and predictable.

And then one day someone barges into a meeting and says, "There is a way we can do *Safety Differently*!" You can't be surprised if you are not immediately met with excitement. To the current team, there is much to give up, much to learn, and much to figure out all over again.

Knowing this group will need some time and attention to build a bridge from the traditional safety effort to doing *Safety Differently* is helpful to building success into the transition process. There is nothing bad, unusual, or abnormal about wanting to hold on to the traditional ideas while learning and understanding the new ideas. It is vital to make this journey to this new set of ideas as logical and welcoming as possible. The organization will want to provide support to the current safety professional staff so they feel supported and informed. This is one group we want to give many learning opportunities. This is the group we want to provide a safe place to practice these new ideas. This is one group we don't want to surprise.

Start where your safety personnel are...not where you want them to be

When helping a group succeed at learning, you must start at the beginning of the concepts. You owe it to your safety team to give them a logical understanding of what doing safety in a different way means to them and your organization. These concepts build upon each other and starting with the fundamentals is important.

Don't assume you can give a quick one-hour overview of a new and different way to manage very important (and often very mature and effective) safety programs. Assigning a book to read or a video to view is helpful but lacks the opportunity to ask questions about this transition. These questions are vital to building expertise and understanding of this new approach.

Some of your team will have been thinking and talking about these ideas for a while, while others of your team will find these ideas stunningly novel, and of course, there will be a group of people somewhere in the middle. Don't assume a level of knowledge that may not be present in your group. Allow time and resources for the group to explore these ideas with the luxury of time and support. Ensure your safety team has all the resources necessary to reach a level of comfort early in the transition, and expertise as this transition goes forward. Remember, these safety professionals will represent the front line of your program. These are the folks that will answer the questions, take the heat, defend the decision, and most importantly ensure your organization is successful in seeing *Safety Differently*.

Build a bridge from the old ideas to the new ideas

The safety professionals should not be made to feel the work that has been done so far with the organization has been misdirected. It is common to compare old thinking to new thinking while discussing the change to a new understanding of safety. This is especially true for organizations that place a lot of emphasis on more traditional safety programs like behavior-based safety, life-saving rule programs, and other worker-directed safety efforts. There will be a belief these programs brought your organization to this place and therefore should not be abandoned for new ideas.[44]

---

[44] The idea that the old programs set the stage for the opportunity to do safety in a different way is not entirely true, but nonetheless it is much easier to think of this change as an addition to the overall historic story of safety in your organization. In reality, the traditional tools have

Don't assume the program you have now is bad and these new ideas are going to be much better. Granted, the new ideas will offer new energy and a new approach for safety, but telling your safety staff to toss out the old and embrace the new may not be as simply done as it is simply said.

It is somewhat offensive to devalue the journey your organization has been on; remember the goal is to move these new ideas successfully from the old, more traditional ideas logically and effectively. There is no advantage to rolling out some type of 'flavor of the month.' Take time to build a case for maturing your safety program to these new ideas. Because of what we have done we now have the opportunity to take our safety program in a different direction.

Always think about attaching new knowledge to the old knowledge. Respectfully help your organization move from where it currently is on its safety journey to where doing *Safety Differently* will move the organization. Be positive in knowing these next steps of this transition will have moments of challenge and many more moments of celebrations. Help your staff and your organization navigate this change positively and successfully. Remember when in doubt; ask your safety team what they will need to be successful. The team will know what is going well and what may need more attention. If you don't know what the team needs, ask them.

---

probably become stagnant and ineffective – part of the reason you are interested in this change is because the old ways are not getting your organization where it needs to go.

The change is in how we see the workers

It is a pretty good bet that your safety team figured out a long time ago the operational expertise in your organization lives with the people who do the work. Doing *Safety Differently* will better align the rest of the organization to this idea and will most likely be a breath of fresh air to the entire safety organization – it helps greatly to bring the rest of the organization in on this knowledge. Helping your organization's safety professional's grasp the different ideas will help clarify what the organization needs the safety team to do differently.

When your organization stops treating workers like they are the problem and starts treating them as if they are the problem-solvers there will be a dramatic change in how the workers think, feel, and engage with the organization. This change will naturally be noticed by the safety professionals in your organization in increased levels of worker engagement, speedy reporting, and an overall sense of shared accountability for operational reliability.

Your safety team will notice two things almost immediately:

1. The levels of trust, communication, shared accountability, and reporting will increase. Worker engagement increases.
2. The safety team's job becomes easier. Knowing more about operations makes you smarter and more effective.

This is all a direct outcome of engaging workers differently. The more you empower workers to own the problems and solutions, the better the safety information is in your organization. Knowing less does not make your safety professionals smarter. The only way to improve the effectiveness of the safety team is for this team to know more. Engaging workers as problem identifiers and problem solvers will give your safety professionals more information about your organization's operations.

A Philosophical Shift from Seeking Deviation to Assuring Capacity

When we talk about engaging safety professionals differently, we are pointing directly at moving your organization's safety effort from an enforcement function to a capacity assurance function. Your safety team has spent hours seeking weaknesses, errors, bad decisions, and violations. One of the traditional roles of a safety professional was to ensure work was not being done wrong.

Now your safety professionals will be allowed to assure work is being done right. One of the most obvious changes is in the relationships built and maintained among the workforce. The traditional role for the safety staff is sometimes seen as the enforcement arm of operations. Doing *Safety Differently* changes the safety professional from fulfilling the role of enforcer to a new role of facilitating what the workers need to do complex, high-consequence work more effectively. Doing *Safety Differently* is quite a remarkable change to any organization.

Engaging safety people in *Safety Differently*

Firstly, continue doing all the things you do now to keep this important group of people happy and motivated. Safety people do hard work for the right reasons and are probably not thanked enough for the work they do. Doing *Safety Differently* has the potential to put more work on an already full plate. When helping your group with a change management strategy, remember to ensure the workers have a voice in what is happening. People actually like change that happens with them in mind. Workers at every level of the organization like to be involved in making changes in their organization; what people hate is the change that happens to them. Don't try to change a group without involving the group in the change. Here are some tips:

- **Start with the fundamentals – build competency on this new way of doing work.** Don't start at the conclusion – start at the beginning and ensure your safety team has the opportunity to develop these ideas so they can better put these ideas into practice. The biggest mistake that can be made is to assume a level of familiarity that is not there.

- **Allow time for discussion and disagreements.** Diversity of thought makes you stronger and makes your transition more effective. It is normal for some initial pushback on these ideas so leave some space in your organization for people to talk about how they are feeling and what they are thinking. Seek places where diverse ideas live in the organization.

- **Know that your safety team members will develop at their own rate.** Not everyone learns at the same rate. Some of your team will jump on these ideas in a short amount of time. Other members of your team may need some more time to think about these ideas. There is no one right way – both of these groups are right and will move at their own rate.

- **Ensure a peer-support group**. Nothing is more comforting than knowing you have some fellow professionals also on the journey. The best resource for difficult questions is the group itself. The combined experience this group represents means there probably is not a question or a problem that some members of the safety team will not have some experience handling.

- **Encourage micro-experimentation.** Encourage safety professionals to try new, worker-engaged ideas in a safe to fail environment. If these new ideas work – repeat them. If these new ideas fail – stop, learn, and move on. The ability to try ideas and gather information about that experiment is how progress is made. The time it takes to try an idea will end up saving you time in the end.

- **Provide protection from the small group that will resist this change.** There will be people who want to submarine this new safety for reasons that never really make much sense when queried. This is normal and sometimes these naysayers will exercise power and force over the safety professionals. Be alert to this idea and be ready to provide some type of protection.

- **Build-in shared accountability for the diffusion of these ideas.** Accountability counts – and nothing is stronger than a sense of shared accountability for the success of any new idea. Talk about the roles that leadership, the workers, and the safety professionals have in doing *Safety Differently*.

- **Tell stories of success during this transition.** Talk about what you have learned. Discuss the events that did not happen because of the work you have done. Be your own press agent. If you don't talk about the success with each other and with the rest of your organization, those stories will not be told. Remember, our organization is used to talking about how safety occasionally fails not how safety normally succeeds.

- **Remember this is fun, exciting and is good for the organization.** Don't lose the joy that comes with making the world a better place. Get caught trying your best.

When the safety team is frustrated, help them

When the safety team is feeling frustrated there is much that still needs to be learned about the transition work being done in your organization. When you feel tension or when you sense a problem it is the time to become instructive and not defensive. The safety team should feel supported, informed and a part of the progress that is being made.

Almost every organization is used to defining safety by counting injuries and accidents. We have been normalized to talking about safety as a set of numbers. Doing *Safety Differently* allows us to talk about safety as a capacity for work that is normally successful. Highlighting this difference alone will serve to engage the safety professionals in an exciting new way.

Discussion questions

1. Why is the way you see workers so fundamental to making any changes that may be needed in the role or orientation of safety people—for example away from being (seen as) the safety police?

2. Is there any evidence of optic compliance, resignation and cynicism around safety rules and policies in your organization? What is responsible for that, you think?

3. What would it take for safety people in your organization to make the philosophical (and practical) shift from seeking deviation to assuring capacity? Who else would need to be on board, and how would that happen?

4. What is the difference between the 'work of safety' and the 'safety of work' in your organization? Are the right people aware of that difference?

5. What stickers, posters or slogans do you have in your organization that all seem to suggest that workers are the problem and that they need to take responsibility for their safety? What might you do about that?

Chapter 6
When you need to help your leaders succeed

> "Those who never change their mind, never change anything."
> - Winston Churchill

Having the opportunity to observe many organizations throughout the world make this change in the way these organizations think about and manage their safety and reliability has allowed us to see some interesting things. We have watched the birth of some incredibly successful ideas and we have seen some missteps that seemed at first glance to be a good idea, but alas did not produce the outcomes imagined. Every organization is on its own voyage of change and the chance to learn from these other organizations is too good to not capture.

We have noticed a trend that is worrying; a trend worth highlighting and pointing out so the next organization on this journey can learn from the last organization. We are trying to fix safety by continuing to try to make the worker be better. In focusing on changing the workers we seem to be missing the actual group in our organization that will best benefit from doing *Safety Differently*. We have targeted the wrong part of the organization to create the change we need. That is a problem we must address, collectively on this journey to doing *Safety Differently*.

Let's talk a bit about this trend and the group we are missing.

Organizations often start this change by training every worker in the organization in some type of mandatory training program. We require workers to attend workshops and watch presentations where we ask them to think about doing the work of safety in a new way. This group is not the correct target for organizational change. We are asking the people who make the machines of work operate amid complex rules, processes, and expectations. We are asking the least influential part of the organization to change the most powerful part of the organization.

Organizations spend a lot of time and effort training their workforces and barely any time at all training the leadership - this trend is especially evident at the most senior leader levels of an organization. Near as we can tell doing a full-blown, major training effort for the workforce is a giant mistake and is an excellent example of spending resources in the wrong place - or not spending the organization's limited time and attention resources in the best way.

It is not that workers don't need to be introduced to the concepts of doing safety in a different way; our workers like and appreciate the opportunity to be a part of the changes that happen in our organizations. It is also true that most workers would not be too disappointed to not have to attend a mandatory training class that rolls out the "new way we are going to be doing our work." Most workers are fine to not have to attend the next safety rollout meeting.

The point is that we train workers because we have easy access to the workers. We don't spend as much time helping leaders be successful. Part of the reason we don't spend the time with the leaders is we simply don't have the same type of access. The hardest time to get is time with leadership. Their time is held as one of the most important organizational resources – and therefore the leaders don't have the opportunity to dig deeper into these concepts and ideas to have a level of expertise around this new set of ideas.

When you look at an organization that is in the process of seeing safety through a new and different lens, the initial push is almost always directed at the workforce. We want every worker to go through some type of workshop where we introduce this list of new ideas, ideas that are very exciting and impactful, to the people who are doing the work. It is not uncommon for an organization to schedule a bunch of workshops and to rotate every worker through some type of required training regimen. As attractive as this idea sounds, and we would guess this idea is attractive because this is the way we have rolled out every other new safety program in what seems like the history of work, this is not a good method for ensuring success.

A giant flavor-of-the-month effort will almost certainly ensure your introduction to these new ideas will be met with skepticism and resistance. The workforce doesn't need a lot of time to process the idea that we blame them for accidents. The workers understand the systems and processes we use to manage work are not written for them to succeed and do more reliable work. The workforce understands the idea that work can't be done the same way every time. Workers are not the problem we are trying to fix.

When we roll out the program to the workforce it is easy to see that we have not shifted our thinking all that much. The organization still believes and is reinforcing these beliefs by the very act of training everyone; the problem is getting the workers to be safer and more reliable. Teaching the people who best understand the problem that there is a problem is not very effective or meaningful. After all, these people cope with these operational complications and pain points every day. This group does not need much (if any) training on these new ideas - and if they did it would be so much better to ask the workers what they need to help make work better. Telling them what they need to do is not helpful. You will never make a group smarter by telling the group how dumb they are.

The group that needs the most, the earliest, the best, and the most basic education on these new ideas is not the workforce. The group that needs the most time is the leadership of the workforce. Leaders are being directly asked to lead differently. Leaders are being asked to not only change the way they lead but also the way they are thinking about the act of leadership.

If we don't help the leaders learn these new ideas, where will they learn?

What seems a much better use of time and energy is to spend a lot of time with the leaders and a short amount of time briefing the workers. The opportunity to do a deeper fundamental discussion with leadership is important but often overlooked because getting the time and attention of a group of already busy leaders is hard to accomplish. Our organizations often give a quick, half-hour overview of what is about to change - and then our organizations are honestly surprised by the lack of depth and experience the leadership level has for these new ideas. You must create time to slowly, (and with the opportunity for leaders to ask questions); build in a depth of knowledge and familiarity with these new ideas and practices. We normally use this rule: Whatever time we budget for the introduction of this new safety philosophy for the workforce, we triple that same amount of time for the leadership level. Amazingly, the three-times factor seems to work extremely well.

It is not like you are shortchanging the workforce. We are fairly certain the workforce won't feel cheated by your effort to streamline their exposure to this new set of ideas. The workforce normally needs less time to understand and give resonance to these ideas. The workers will see the results of the new approach almost immediately and will, most likely, feel a sense of relief. Telling the workforce the change is happening is important; giving them every detail of the change is not as important to the workers. They will judge the success of this change in actions, not in words on the screen.

Leaders will need time to think about and practice some of these ideas. These ideas will seem very new and perhaps a bit risky to them on first exposure. We are asking these leaders to respond earlier and differently than we have traditionally asked them to react in the past. We are both philosophical and operationally moving the leadership effort towards managing the capacity to do high-risk work effectively and that means we are moving the leadership efforts away from the normal and comfortable outcome management model.

Don't underestimate how big this change is for your leaders - it is a big change.

Expect your leadership team to have a long adjustment period to this new way of responding. Expect this change to happen slower than you wish it would happen because it will be slower than you wish. Expect leaders to fall back to their old ways once in a while. Remember the old agrarian adage: "When thunder cracks the horse will always want to run back to the barn." Mostly, be patient and help serve as a sounding board and a guide as your organization moves forward. There is hope, however, as leaders get more and more comfortable, this change becomes easier and more effective.

The key to success is almost entirely held by providing the opportunity for your leaders to become experts in this new way of thinking. Allow these leaders the chance to make these ideas their own. Time and time again, when looking at organizations that have not had very much success in changing the course of their safety program, the problem has been in the leadership of the organization not being given the time or the information to understand what these leaders need to do differently. It is not that the leaders can't change (for the most part leaders are quite good at change), but is more that these leaders have not been given the fundamental information to understand what they need to do, differently, in this new paradigm.

We assume that leaders have the same exposure to and comfort with these new ideas as the safety team may have. We know that is not possible. If we don't create an opportunity for leaders to learn these new ideas it will not happen magically – If we don't take the time to facilitate leadership success, we will not have successful leaders.

> *You never know what will trigger a shift in thinking in a leader. Different people realize this new way of thinking in different ways. Knowing what will be the catalyst for new thinking in any learner, not just at the leadership level, is a mystery that we are constantly trying to discover.*

We were invited to take part in a meeting to address a series of near-catastrophic events involving dropped objects. The organization was very motivated to address this problem seriously. The entire meeting was spent talking about how this organization would have a global stand-down to emphasize the seriousness of these dropped objects, then the organization would combine a behavior-based safety program with a poster/sign/sticker campaign directed at the tool-pushers and this would all be reinforced with a mandatory training program delivered at the worksite for all three shifts. The organization was talking about millions of dollars to tell the workers to stop dropping stuff.

Finally, we were asked to discuss what we thought about this problem. We mustered up great levels of respect and started our part of the discussion by making a bold and broad-stroke statement.

"Every dropped object is a mistake. Mistakes are unintentional – workers don't choose to make (or not make) mistakes – mistakes are normal and never causal. Asking workers to not drop tools and equipment from height feels like you are taking action, but in reality, is an enormous was of time, energy and money."

The room was silent – very silent.

The big boss said, "That can't be right. That just can't be right. How on earth can you say that?"

> *Our response was, "Every dropped object has to be a mistake. If the worker chooses to drop the object – if the worker dropped the object on purpose that is not a dropped object. We have a word for objects dropped on purpose and that work is throwing. If you have workers who are throwing objects then you suck at personnel selection – you are hiring the wrong people."*
>
> *It was at that very moment the Senior Vice President realized the new thinking that doing Safety Differently would require. That senior leader has become one of the most informed and well-studied leaders in his company, perhaps in the world.*
>
> *His company is now deliberately building capacity in all the work they do.*

You never know what will change the thinking of a leader. You can never know what story or comment will break through the years and years of the traditional approach to managing safety. You should never be hesitant to have the same conversation many, many times. Steady reinforcement of new thinking in a safe and effective way is how change happens – but this change won't happen if your organization does not deliberately create space for leaders to learn, expand and practice these new ideas. Never give up – keep the faith and know that long journeys have many steps.[45]

---

[45] This idea is taken from Lao Tzu – a journey of a thousand miles begins with a single step and that step could be a life defining (organizational-redefining) beginning to a new way of thinking.

Spend your limited resource allotment on setting leadership up to be successful

You have a limited amount of time and money to do the important work you do. It is also true you have limited numbers of times you can attract and hold the attention of your organization's leaders - both physically and intellectually. Use these scarce opportunities wisely and make the best out of your very limited chance to have a direct and meaningful impact on leadership. Knowing this is an almost sacred opportunity is a lot of pressure on you, but also is an excellent way to know where to best prioritize your efforts. As a rule, we test almost all the change decisions by asking one important question; "Will this effort (training, book clubs, travel) create an environment where the leaders of the organization will be successful in guiding and using these new ideas and concepts?" In short, will this set leaders up to be knowledgeable, prepared, unsurprised, and effective in doing the important work of *Safety Differently*?

These questions will serve you well. Creating tools and resources for leaders to know what to do differently is extremely important. Giving leaders a safe place to practice these ideas is vital. Using safe-to-fail micro-experiments and then understanding and discussing the outcomes of these trial balloons gives leaders confidence in moving forward when the road gets a bit rockier and there is a real consequence to their actions.

Knowing they are not alone on this change journey is also extremely valuable to helping create an environment where change can be successful. Building a community of leaders, a peer group, if you will, to provide support and education, is vital to creating success.

When leaders push back - become instructive, not offended

It is normal for leaders to push back on these ideas. Perhaps the most asked question is the question of accountability - leaders want to know how they can hold workers accountable for the failures that happen in the leader's organization - that discussion is a good one to have, but for this discussion let's discuss how we can make a leader's discomfort with these new ideas a bit more palatable, a bit more comfortable, which will lead to better long-term adoption of these ideas.

Let's start with an important assumption: A leader should be pushing back on these ideas.

These ideas, although not really meant to be direct criticisms of the organization's leadership activities for the last several years, are going to be a pretty strong dose of reality. In a way, when we discuss the deliberate leadership decisions that have been made in the past and will be made differently in the future, we are holding the organization up to a big, ugly mirror (the kind with magnification). We are forcing the organization to think about the potential negative impacts past decisions have had on the current and future state of the organization.

If your organization's leadership does not push back, you are not effectively communicating these ideas to the group. Expect leaders to question these new ideas against years of corporate leadership expectations to provide strong command and control, to punish the guilty, and to always push the blame to the sharp end of the organization. Of course, leaders are going to question why this change is happening now - and these leaders have every right to ask this question. Be ready for the pushback and know that when the pushback happens this is what the birth of a new idea looks and sounds like when it is happening.

Try to remember when we are asking a leader to do work in a very different way; this leader is being exposed to an entirely new level of personal and professional risk. This type of change can and often is a bit scary and that is not only OK but also pretty predictable and normal. Heighten your sensitivity to the individual needs leaders have. Push, but push them with love and support. Take these leaders from where they are to where the organization best needs them to go - but know this is a journey to new leadership, not a switch that can be flicked in a half-hour meeting.

What about looking at how badly we managed safety in the past?

We don't think much is gained by rehashing the past much beyond the idea that the past was an example of one way of thinking while the more important use of time and energy is gained by using this same path as the starting place for changing operational understanding of safety and reliability. Reopening old cases, like reopening old wounds, only seems to cause pain in retrospect and offers very little by the way of ways to make the past organizational responses have any different or better outcomes.

However, in the same voice, we would add that the ability to look to the past and learn and understand where the organization was (or currently is) is quite important. This type of retrospective learning is best done in small, controlled ways allowing for learning to happen without causing leaders to look bad - this is a tricky opportunity - but none the less an opportunity that has much to offer if this assessment learning is done well, done with respect, and done with the most positive intentions.

Revisiting old decisions about blame and accountability will produce a new set of problems with the workforce, the union if you have exposure there, the idea of fairness, and the simple fact there is a new way to understand what failed as opposed to who failed. The ability to learn from the past is rich, however, the cost of this learning is something that must be monitored carefully and with great sensitivity to the context of these decisions. Viewing any action in retrospect will always make you smarter, but you must ask at what cost. Simply drawing a line and saying, "From this point forward our organization will change the way we learn and respond to events," is in so many ways much cleaner and much less culturally dangerous.

We must start the process of changing the way our organization thinks about safety and reliability with the identification of what the leadership is currently thinking and doing to help the leadership move to a much better operational place. Knowing your starting place is found at the exact current state of the organizational leadership function is a rather comforting bit of knowledge. Knowing this starting place also greatly improves your ability to successfully help these leaders begin the process of shifting their basic assumptions about how to lead a complex organization in the midst of constant variability. Identifying and using this starting place allows you and your team to carefully craft and tailor the message specifically to the organization and where the organization is currently positioned on the arc of this change journey.

Having and using this knowledge is vital in helping leaders succeed in the new ways you are asking them to think and respond.

Emphasize the things the organization is doing that are currently effective and thoughtful (there will be many to be sure) and discuss the places where the organization has the most opportunity for dramatic and effective improvement. None of that information is possible if you don't understand where the organization is currently situated. Knowing where the organization is and starting at that point allows the change to attach to the old ways while at the same time introducing the new ways of thinking, acting and leading.

Remember leadership action and behaviors are directly influenced by the organizations' systems and processes just as that is true for the workers these leaders lead. One way to build leadership success is to change the information that is reported up the chain. When you tell leaders only the stories of failures in their organizations, after a while, the leaders will get the impression that only failure happens. We must change the dialogue we have with leadership in order to reinforce the new way of thinking and managing the organization. One of the best examples of this change of narrative to reflect the doing of *Safety Differently* is a company that added one question to the event-reporting document that was sent to the senior leadership every week.

This organization realized the importance of changing the discussion so it was determined they would add one additional question to this report. The question that was added was: "Did the presence of a safeguard change the consequence of this event? If so, how? If not, what safeguard should be in place and functioning for this specific work?"

This one simple addition had a very strong positive effect on the way the leaders thought about these reports. The most important benefit is this additional information in turn changed the questions the leaders asked about the report. All told, the leadership questions almost exclusively focused on the safeguards and not on the workers involved. This experiment was an incredible success.

When you need to help leaders to succeed remember these ideas

Here are the vital touchstones to helping your organization's leadership be successful, which in turn will better ensure your organizational change to seeing *Safety Differently* is successful. This list is from our observations and is probably not complete, but does serve to highlight some of the most important factors necessary for ensuring your leadership is supported and will be best prepared to succeed.

> 1. Meet your leadership team where they are in this process. Don't assume leaders already know this information – most likely leaders will not have been exposed

to many of these ideas.

2. Help your leaders move their definition of safety from the old view, safety as an outcome, to the newer view of seeing safety as a capacity. This seemingly simple change is fundamental to every other change that will happen.

3. Build sufficient time for presenting these new ideas, discussing these new ideas, and pushing back on these new ideas. Don't allow the fear of a busy schedule to shorten the amount of time you spend in creating successful change. No matter how hard your leadership team will try to shorten the schedule, and they will try to shorten the schedule, staying true to the rule of more time being the better option.

4. Allow the opportunity to practice this new way of responding to operational failure. Use case studies, other peer leaders from other organizations, and discussion time to help build competency in responding differently.

5. Build expertise at the leadership level – create a path for your leaders to be experts in this new way of thinking. Tell these leaders the organization needs them to be experts in operational reliability and safety.

6. Help recognize and reinforce leadership peer groups within your organization–

your leader's co-workers are not the people they lead; your leadership's co-workers are their fellow leaders. Change is less scary when change is shared among peers. There is strength (and confidence) in numbers.

7. Tell stories of success – don't underestimate the power of the many small successes that are happening in your organization all the time.

8. And finally, know that your leaders will move forwards and backwards in leading the organization towards this new way of thinking and responding – it takes a while to change years of experience.

One of us was talking with a group of leaders. They were looking at a picture of so-called 'shared space' in road traffic: the kind of place where there are no traffic signs, no lights, no designations, lines or anything else painted on the road – just a uniform square (or open space) for everyone to mingle and figure it out together. That is very much how roads used to be if you look at pictures from the beginning of the twentieth century.

"Hang on a minute," said one leader. "What if we were to do that?"

We said, "Do what?"

The leader replied: "Take everything out. All the safety stuff we have put in. All the top-down rules, the signs, the checklists, the procedures."

Others were looking at him.

"As an experiment," he continued. "See what happens. See how people create safety when they're left alone."

It took eighteen months to convince only some of his fellow executives, but also the various regulators who oversee different aspects of their operations. And of course, we had to design the experiment, do a pilot trial, get unions on board, and explore a way to randomly assign conditions to groups of comparable sites. We also had to make the experiment 'safe-to-fail.' We inserted the assurance of being able to pull the plug on the whole thing at any time, and quickly revert to the old system of top-down safety controls. If ever we got the slightest hunch that risk was going up because of the experiment, or worse, that someone had got hurt in one of the experimental conditions, we'd call it quits immediately.

It wasn't as if nobody was getting hurt under the old system. People were. Incident and injury rates had flat lined for a while and were now on the rise.

What did people think about this, the people who worked on the frontlines? As you might have expected, the old system of centralized safety was largely despised. No worker thought that safety people knew what they were talking about, and they were convinced that none of the bureaucratic work-of-safety they were forced to comply with had anything to do with improving the safety of their work. There were set requirements for safety committees, safety meetings, and safety boards, safety procedures, safety notices. Nobody took notice. Of any of it. One worker told us: "I don't think about safety. I just follow the rules and do as I'm told." Getting on a safety committee was not based on merit or skills or knowledge. It was sometimes seen as a punishment or as a welcome (though in content entirely useless) reprieve from other work.

It sure was time for a change.

But changing everything overnight, across the company, was seen as too bold, stupid, or dangerous. And where was the evidence that another approach might work better?

This is where the micro-experiment comes in.[46] *It's a great way to engage leaders in the ideas of doing Safety Differently because it offers up a part of their organization to create the data that another approach may be better (for them as well!).*

---

[46] The idea for this 'micro-experiment,' formally known as 'the Woolworths experiment' comes from Sidney Dekker. The experimental protocol and study execution was conducted largely by Michelle Oberg, a doctoral student in the Safety Science Innovation Lab at the time of the Woolworths Experiment. Martin O'Neill was the senior leader at Woolworths who championed the Woolworths Experiment. He has been fielding calls regularly from colleagues at other organizations, asking him how in the world he did it. Countless men and women

A micro-experiment is a safe-to-fail, small-scale project, using the company's workplaces and workforce. The aim is to explore and test doing Safety Differently, for example by taking out a procedure or removing duplicate paperwork. In this case, it involved taking out pretty much everything related to safety. The intention was to do this at a small group of sites, under controlled conditions, compared to other, similar sites, where we either did something different or changed nothing at all.

The only things we could not take out were fire exit signs, as they are federally mandated. And there were a few more items like them. The idea of a micro-experiment is that it generates the kind of credible, internally validated data that an organization can use to build some confidence that a different approach to safety might work for them.

So, we devised three conditions:

- *Take everything out. This condition, which we formally called the 'local ownership condition,' was the one in which we removed all the safety processes, procedures, checklists and rules that were not specifically required by state or federal law. In this condition, we wanted to create completely open conditions for grass-roots safety to germinate and grow. We took everything out, made no suggestions about what to do instead, and left the stores with only one rule: 'don't hurt anyone.'*

at Woolworths were instrumental in making the micro-experiment happen, as well as stakeholders at the regulator and other partner organizations. You can watch the experiment in the free documentary film '*Safety Differently*' on YouTube.

- *Take everything out and retrain according to Safety Differently. This condition, which we formally called the 'ownership and engagement condition', was driven by deliberate change management, which included training sessions for store workers and managers. These were modeled on the ideas of Safety Differently: see people as a resource to harness, not as a problem to control. Don't tell people what to do but ask what they need to be successful, and stop counting negatives as a measure of your progress. Instead, identify and support the positive capacities in your people and teams that make things go well. We wanted this condition in there to see whether there were any radical differences between how people organized safety for themselves when left entirely to their own devices, and how they did so when actively instructed or inspired along new lines. In this condition, too, workers and managers were empowered to take out what they didn't think was useful.*

- *Control condition. This condition was literally our control. It involved a group of stores that were comparable to the stores in the other two conditions, but we changed nothing in them. They kept doing what they had been doing. Head office stayed in control of safety. It kept sending down its safety packs and expecting compliance in return. Managers or workers were not given any more leeway.*

We randomly identified ten sites to assign to each condition, for a total of 30. This was of course a bit tricky. We needed to avoid 'picking the winners' for the first two conditions (which I'll collectively call the 'ownership' conditions). That would have been easy. In conversations with leaders, we quickly learned that some managers were known to be willing to try new things, to be naturally more open to new ideas, interested in their employees and accessible for them. It would have been easy to seek those out and assign them to the ownership conditions, as that would surely lead to success. But it would mess up the experiment, because how could we fairly compare across the conditions if we put the presumed winners in the conditions we wanted to win, and left the more hopeless places and managers to the control condition?

The thirty sites had to start from the same place. And they pretty much did. Then we randomly assigned the three groups of ten stores to the three conditions. The experiment started the day we took everything out of the sites in the first condition and started training people in the second condition. It finished a year later. There was no loss of data during the year of the experiment, as all sites stayed with us throughout.

Bigger Worries

Of course, there were some concerns beyond the sheer design of the experiment. If there is collective representation, for instance, then what do unions say when you start 'experimenting' with worker safety? Interestingly, our experiences show that the responses are quite diverse, or even ambivalent. On the one hand, unions are rightly concerned when you announce you are going to take away the reasonable employer-provided protections that seem to keep their workers safe.

And what about the organization's lawyers, how do they look at this? Again, our experience was that there is no substitute for sitting down with stakeholders, including lawyers, and being open-minded about their concerns. We rationally went through all the pros and cons of changing these things about work. With reasonable safeguards in place and a limited scope that specifically aims to improve how an organization does its business and protects its workers, there are few obstacles. This went for regulators as well. We found that the ones who were most closely concerned about workplace health and safety had also begun to understand that doing more of the same was not going to generate different results. They, too, were keen to hear new ideas and explore different ways to improve safety results.

Results

When given the opportunity, people gladly throw off the yoke of bureaucracy and compliance. 19 out of 20 stores (a full 95%) from the two ownership conditions immediately ceased compliance activities mandated by the corporate safety department. They all agreed that these things added no value, and didn't impact safety outcomes. A store manager commented: "I think that removing the administrative tasks has inspired the team to be driven to look at safety in a different light. Instead of a chore, it is now more enjoyable: they look, observe and engage in what matters, day to day."

And indeed, the store manager's role changed as well. They no longer performed the role of overseer and auditor. Instead of chasing workers for dates and signatures on meaningless paperwork, they found that they were spending more time with people—listening to what mattered to them, discovering the daily obstacles and challenges that stood in the way of creating success. Workers, in turn, found managers to be much more responsive to their concerns. Local ownership meant something. When we surveyed workers on their perceptions of leadership, those in our two ownership conditions rated their managers higher on the ability to empower individuals and enhance skills and self-sufficiency than anywhere else in the organization.

Interestingly, sites and managers in the ownership conditions also became more assertive in requesting help from the head office. Now that they had more ownership for safety, and more engagement locally, they didn't hesitate to make their needs and demands known to those who were tasked with supporting or supplying them. Some were bemused that it took an experiment run by a university to restore or invigorate their internal organizational links and relationships. And sites in the ownership conditions saw more initiative across the board, for example by introducing better procedures or better tools.

Freedom In a Frame

These are not complex interventions, of course. But the results can be amazing. In the second ownership condition, there was a reduction in the number of lost-time injuries (if we still wanted to see that as a relevant measure: many people did). It was interesting for us to see that the number and diversity of initiatives (like bringing in or adopting new tools to perform tasks) were greater in the second ownership condition. Only setting people free was not enough: people need some inspiration of what can be done, of what they can potentially achieve, they need some knowledge and active empowerment through examples of what others have achieved in similar circumstances. They also need that sense of a frame, of something shared and a larger purpose that sits around their local initiatives.

Decluttering compliance and bureaucracy is a good start. But the second ownership condition showed that engaging people actively in a different way of doing safety and giving them the freedom and autonomy to pick and choose and develop what they want is an even more powerful combination. The trap is that any guidance on how to do Safety Differently can become yet another kind of authority, another kind of top-down intervention, and another way of telling people what to do. We avoided this as much as we could, by leaving the actual development of safety work and other interventions to people themselves.

A Whoopee Prize

The jewel in the crown of the experiment came toward the end. One of the sites in the second ownership (take everything out) condition was awarded the company's annual safety prize. The committee awarding the prize wasn't aware of the experiment but must have liked what they saw, and the results it produced. We can't say for sure that the store won the prize because it was in the 'take everything out and retrain' condition. But we can say for sure that being in that condition didn't hurt their chances of winning it. That should be reassuring to anyone wanting to try a similar micro-experiment.

But wasn't this all caused by the Hawthorne effect? The Hawthorne effect refers to organizational research originally conducted during the 1920s and 1930s at the Hawthorne Works, an electric factory in Illinois. In those experiments, researchers wanted to know whether worker productivity changed with variations in lighting, break times, and working hours. It changed, for sure, but not with any clear correlation to the variations in whatever the researchers were manipulating in the workplace. Productivity went up across the board. When the researchers packed up and left, productivity slumped again. Researchers concluded that worker productivity goes up simply because you're paying attention to workers, and because you show interest in their situation. A little humanity goes a long way. But it does create a potential confound in studies such as this micro-experiment.

The way we dealt with that was to be scrupulous about how much attention we gave to, and how much time we spent with workers and store managers across all conditions. So even the stores in the condition in which nothing was changed, where the old regime was still in place, got as many visits and conversations from us as the other two. In this way, we kept the amount of attention given to workers constant across all three conditions, thereby spreading any Hawthorne effect out overall conditions equally and thus leaving them comparable. This gave us confidence that the change in leadership perceptions and safety results in the two ownership conditions were related to our safety anarchism changes, and not just because we were there.

Can you do your own micro-experiment?

So, what do you need so that you can conduct your own micro-experiment? Before we answer that question, just consider this: In many organizations, it may not be smart to call a micro-experiment an 'experiment,' as it invokes fears and uncertainties about 'experimenting,' about trying out new ideas, methods or activities that play fast and loose with peoples safety. For risk-averse managers or boards, it is probably less problematic to call it a 'project.' Organizations always have projects going on. It can then even designate someone to be the 'project manager.' This should not, however, detract from the rigorous scientific design of the experiment that runs under the label of 'project.' It is this design, after all, and the strict comparability across conditions, that allows leadership to draw valid and reliable conclusions about doing *Safety Differently* in its own organization.

Here's what you do:

1. Find two or more groups (sites, teams, locations) that are comparable because they do similar work and have a similar make-up. To the extent that you can control it, make sure that these groups will remain relatively stable for the duration of the experiment (e.g., no management shakeups, no radical changes of leadership). If there are such changes along the way, you may have a harder time attributing any results to what you did, as opposed to what was done to the group by those other factors.

2. Study what you can change or take out. Is there unnecessary bureaucratic clutter? Is there overlap? A typical case of overlap would be procedures that a contractor uses, which do almost the same as those the lead organization uses, but people working for the contractor (which is working for the lead organization) have to do both. Are there rules that nobody believes in? You can find this out by asking what people consider to be the stupidest thing they have to do every day to be allowed to work on a particular site or project. It's a great question to ask, and you'll surely get enlightening answers.

3. Do a small pilot. This might involve just talking to people, testing your idea through a thought experiment, or testing it live with a group of people. You can learn a lot from these small pilots (e.g., you might learn that

the thing you wanted to take out is not at all what frustrates people the most).

4. Reserve the time to let the change(s) take effect. Don't think you can do a micro-experiment inside of a few weeks, though you might see some immediate effects (as we observed in the micro-experiment above: the previously mandatory safety work was abandoned as soon as they were no longer required in the ownership conditions). Other effects will take more time to become visible.

5. Measure the changes. You can do that by using safety indicators and measures you are already using, but you might also want to think about additional measures to take that are more positive than that (e.g., leadership perception, empowerment and locus of control, happiness at work). Think about what you've read in chapter 1: what capacities are needed to make things go well?

6. Collate the findings, celebrate the successes and communicate them to others in the organization, so they are inspired to take your experiences onboard. They may even be inspired to do their micro-experiments to innovate and improve an area of their work.

Remember, a micro-experiment is powerful in part because it involves data generated by your own organization. It's not just an idea or a belief: it is evidence that another way of working is possible — and very possibly better.

Sustaining these new ideas and newly changed leaders

One of the most important (and most uncomfortable) things we have learned while doing the type of work we all do, is progress is not permanent. Progress is not permanent. We always thought that once an organization became enlightened, the organization would only move forward and become better and better. After all, once you begin to see the world in this new way it is pretty difficult to go back to the old ways of seeing the world, or so we thought.

Or at least we hoped that would be the case. Progress towards improvement is a fragile and dainty state of being - which can be easily lost if conditions and personalities align in a 'just right' way.

Organizations ebb and flow, they get better and they slide backwards. Just because we have done great work getting a senior leadership team to change the way they react to events in the everyday occurrence of doing work, we are not assured this change is cemented into the foundation of our organization in some type of permanent way. We, all of us, are just one new executive away from having to start again at the very beginning.

We know that is uncomfortable to highlight, but we will not get the desired change we need by ignoring the fact our job of challenging, educating, and coaching will never go away. We will always be completing the process of changing and organization - because the process of changing and organization never stops happening.

This is the point of building-in sustainable philosophical shifts in organizations - there does not seem to be one magic action that makes an idea sustain past the current people who are holding these ideas for the organization. That seems disappointing, and probably is a hard thing to reckon with both emotionally and intellectually, but in reality, the idea that we must continuously work on understanding safety and reliability in a new and better way in order to keep these ideas alive and well is a great opportunity to continuously improve upon these ideas, refining and making the methods for doing work in a complex world better and better.

What makes an idea sustainable? What makes an idea stick to an organization beyond the personalities that steer and direct these ideas on a daily basis? In short, the answer must lie in the idea that the organization is better because the organization is managing complex work in a way that is clearly more effective. There is nothing better to keep an idea alive than the story of how the use of this new idea creates success stories.

Change is best understood by seeing how change makes our organization different.

Saying change is found by looking for change sounds obvious (and it is really obvious); what is amazing is that many organizations look for a change in places where change is difficult to notice any observable impact on the operation. This only gets more difficult when the change you seek is the absence of an event – it is hard to measure something that hasn't happened.

Change is best understood by seeing how change makes an organization different. This may seem painfully obvious. It *is* painfully obvious, but you won't be surprised to know that almost all organizations are aligned and rigged in such a way as to reinforce the status quo - to keep things the same as much as possible. This idea that the organization will actively work against change is a very real part of any good sustainability strategy - and in reality, probably the most important part of keeping these ideas alive.

We must maintain these new ideas in practice by continually evaluating the ability of this new approach to create a different and better outcome for the organization. We can support leadership and sustain this change.

Building these new ideas into our other practices, processes and procedures has great value as well. Doing *Safety Differently* will eventually find its way to doing operations differently. Seeing work differently has a way of making an organization better.

Discussion questions

1. When it comes to doing safety differently, has your organization's leadership been largely missing from that conversation? Or have they been driving it? What are the reasons for that, you think?

2. How can you support your leaders in making these safety differently ideas their own? Have they pushed back on them before? What happened then?

3. Can you think of a viable micro-experiment in your organization or unit? What would you compare or test, how would you do that, and what would you hope to find or demonstrate?

4. What needs to be in place or change in your organization to make safety differently not only a viable, but sustainable way of doing safety?

5. What have you missed in this book? What would you like, or need, to discuss more of?

About the Authors

Sidney Dekker (Ph.D. Ohio State University, USA, 1996) is Professor and Director of the Safety Science Innovation Lab at Griffith University in Brisbane, Australia, and Professor at the Faculty of Aerospace Engineering at Delft University in the Netherlands.

Sidney has lived and worked in seven countries across four continents and won worldwide acclaim for his groundbreaking work in human factors and safety. He popularized the *New View* of human error in safety in 2001 with his first *Field Guide* and coined the term *Safety Differently* in 2012, which has since turned into a global movement for change. *Safety Differently* encourages organizations to declutter their bureaucracy and provide people freedom-in-a-frame to make things go well—and to offer compassion, restoration and learning when they don't. An avid piano player and pilot, he has been flying the Boeing 737 for an airline on the side.

Sidney is the bestselling author of, most recently: *Foundations of Safety Science*; *The Safety Anarchist*; *The End of Heaven*; *Just Culture*; *Safety Differently*; *The Field Guide to Understanding 'Human Error'*; *Second Victim*; *Drift into Failure*; *Patient Safety* and his latest: *Compliance Capitalism*. He has co-directed the documentaries *Safety Differently*, 2017; *Just Culture*, 2018, *The Complexity of Failure*, 2018, and *Do Safety Differently*, 2019. Stanford has ranked Sidney among the world's top 2% most influential scientists: his work has some 15000 citations and an *h*-index of 53. More at sidneydekker.com

Todd Conklin (Ph.D. University of New Mexico, USA, 2001) retired from Los Alamos National Laboratory and lives a life of leisure and non-responsibility filled joy in Santa Fe, New Mexico in the United States. Conklin spends his time now helping organizations, both large and small, shift their focus from the traditional view of safety to Doing Safety Differently.

Todd spent almost 30 years at Los Alamos National Laboratory as a Senior Advisor for Organizational and Safety Culture. Los Alamos National Laboratory is one of the world's foremost research and development laboratories; Dr. Conklin has been working on the Human Performance program for most of his career. It is in this fortunate position where he enjoys the best of both the academic world and the world of safety in practice.

Todd holds a Ph.D. in organizational behavior and was fortunate to study with Everett Rodgers, author of the important work *Diffusion of Innovation*. It was during this time that Conklin became interested in how organizations diffuse new ideas in to their traditional organization.

Todd has written several books: *Simple Revolutionary Acts, Pre-Accident Investigations, Better Questions, Workplace Fatalities, When the Worst Thing Happens, The 5 Principles of Human Performance*, and most recently, *Do Safety Differently*.

The **Pre Accident Podcast** is heard twice weekly and has millions of downloads. This podcast is an ongoing discussion about doing safety differently and enjoys international recognition by safety professionals, workers, and leaders in highly reliable organizations.

Todd speaks all over the world to executives, groups and work teams who are interested in better understanding the relationship between the workers in the field and the organization's systems, processes, and programs. He has brought these systems to major corporations around the world. Conklin practices these ideas not only in his own workplace, but also in the event investigations at other workplaces around the world. Conklin defines safety at his workplace like this: "Safety is the ability for workers to be able to do work in a varying and unpredictable world."

Made in the USA
Monee, IL
27 April 2025